ZIPZAP BRAIN SNAP

Meet the Amygdala

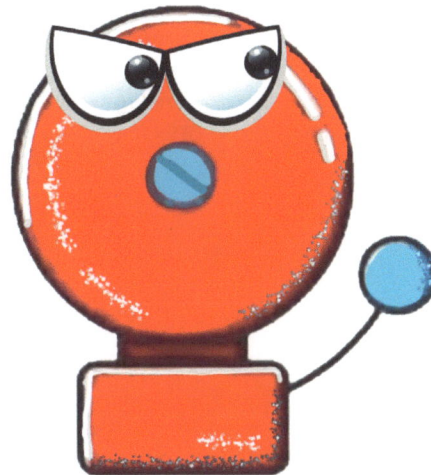

Shakti A. Burke

First edition KDP 2021 (revised)

ISBN 978-0-6484796-6-6

Published by Joyfulmind Wellbeing
Maclean NSW Australia
www.joyfulmind.net.au

joyfulmind108@gmail.com

Designed on the canva platform
www.canva.com

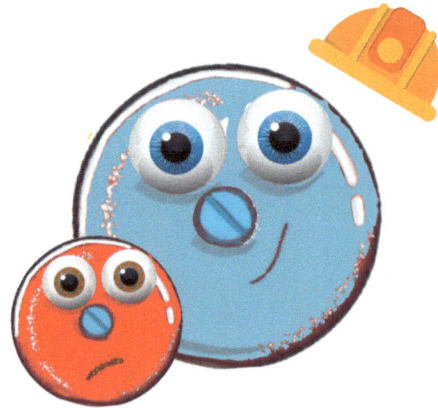

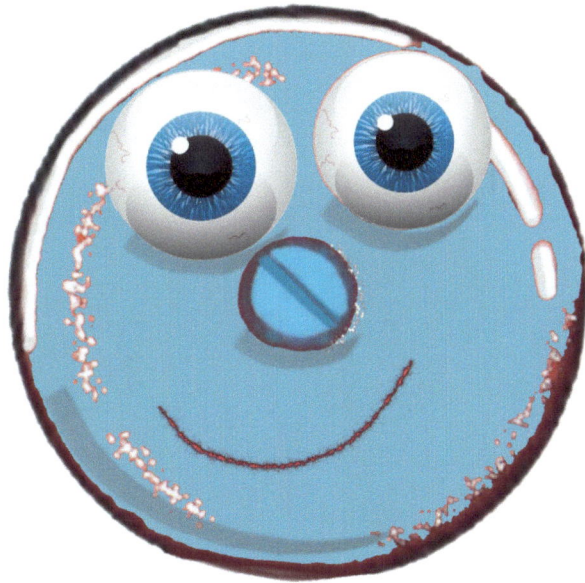

joyfulmind.net.au

1

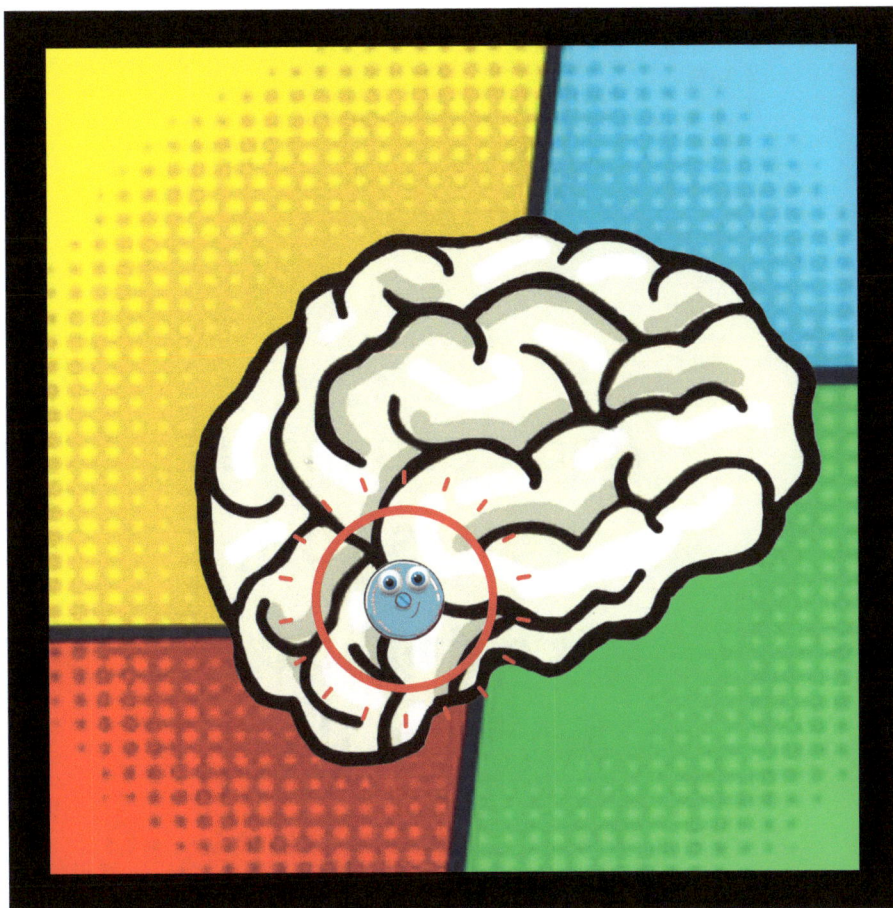

1.
Amygdala

Deep inside my brain

And deep inside
yours too,

is a tiny little
pea-sized thing
with one big job to do.

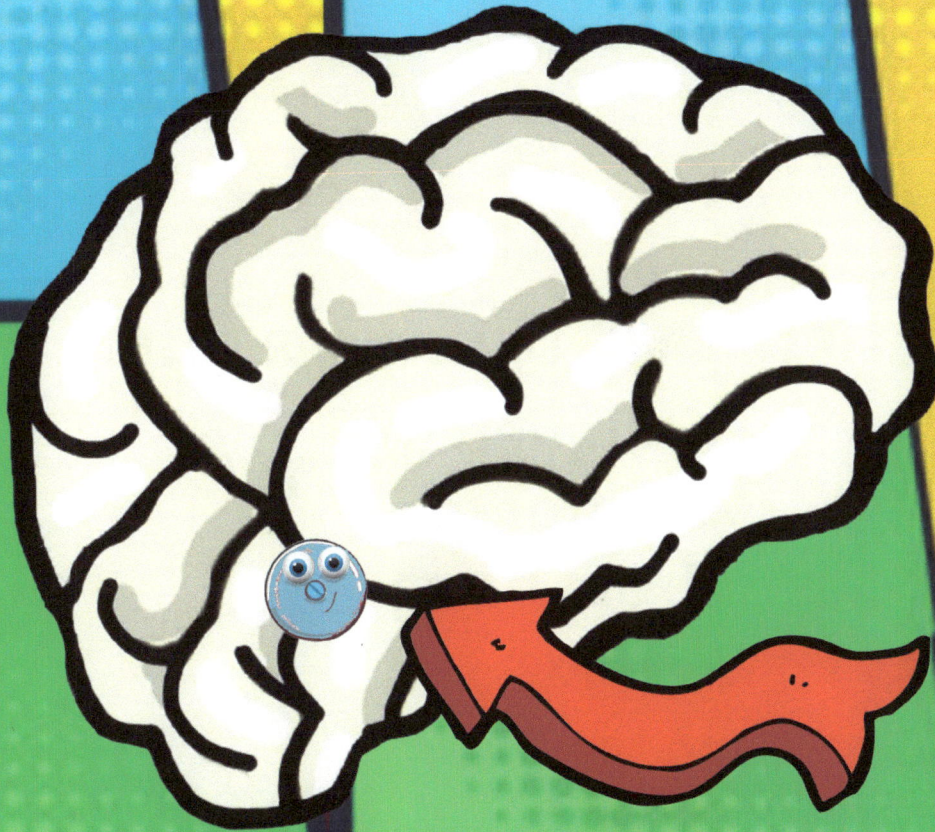

a-mig-da-la

It's designed to keep me safe,
assigned to
shelter me
from harm

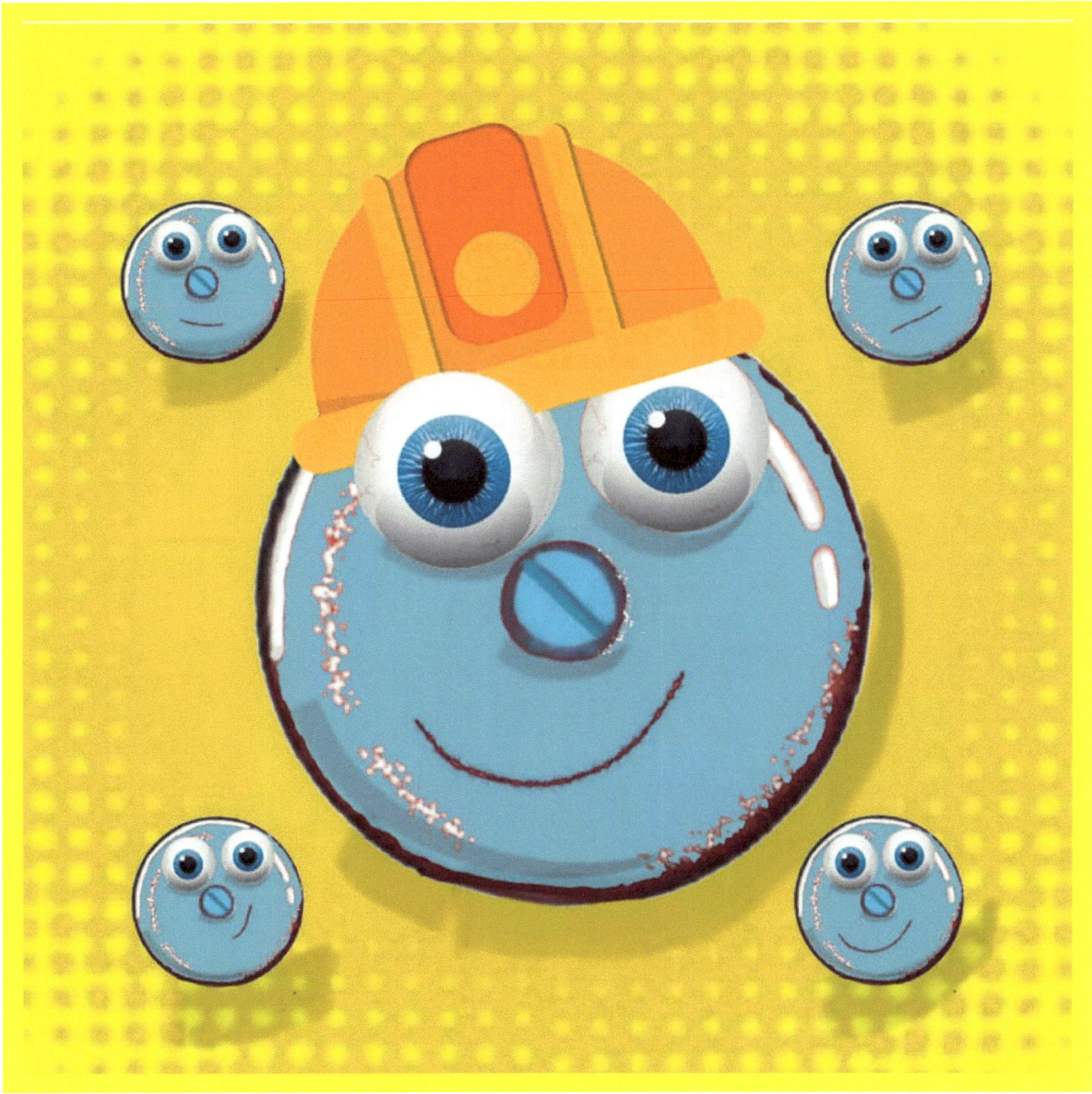

When danger strikes
it peaks and spikes
and sounds a
big alarm.

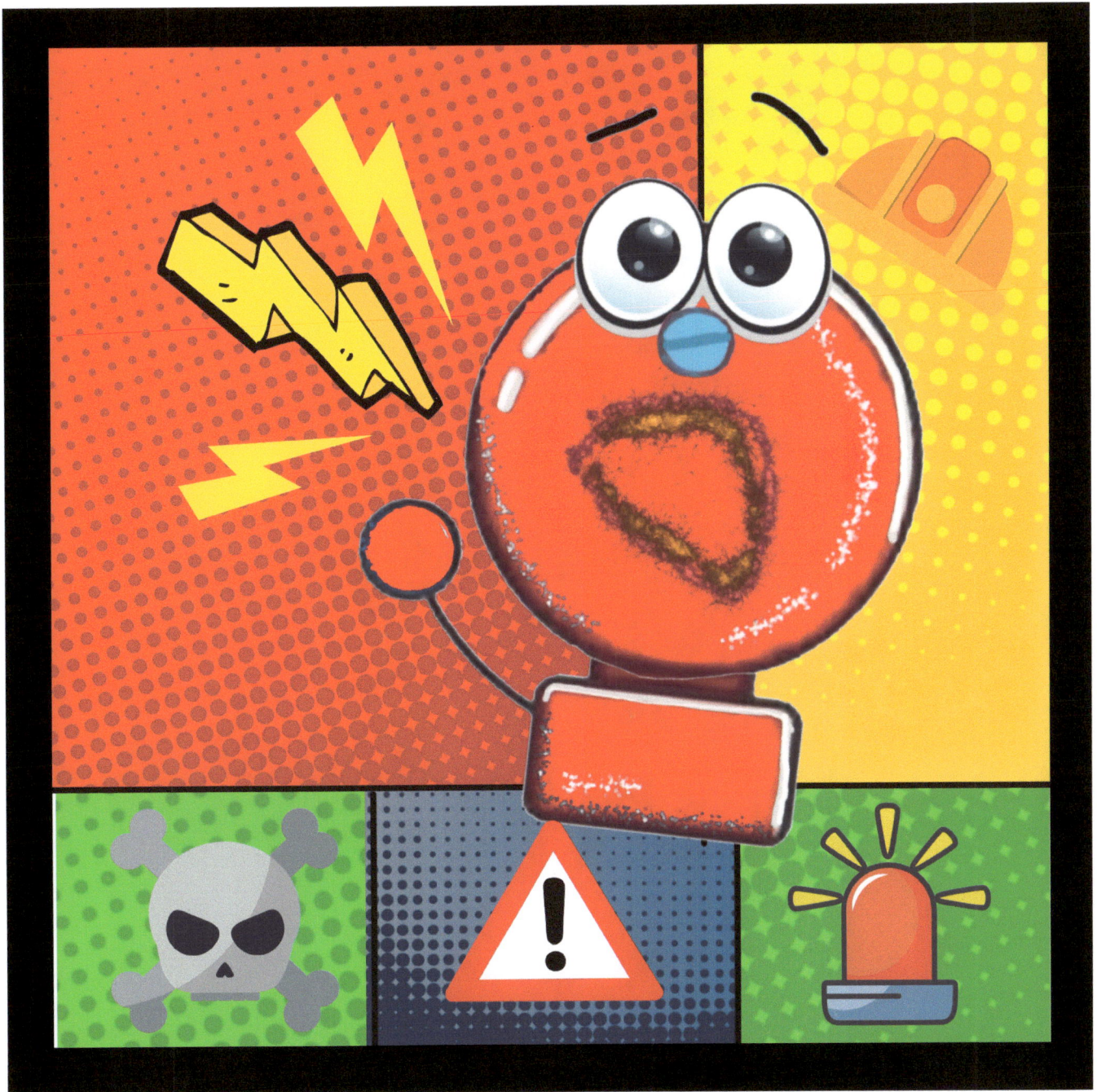

AMIG AMIG AMIG DA

la la la la laa-la

this tiny little bit of brain has got me in its pow-a

ZIP ZAP

BRAIN SNAP

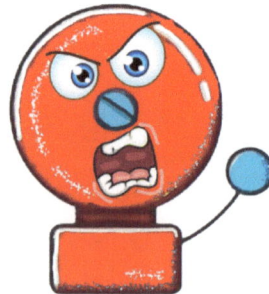

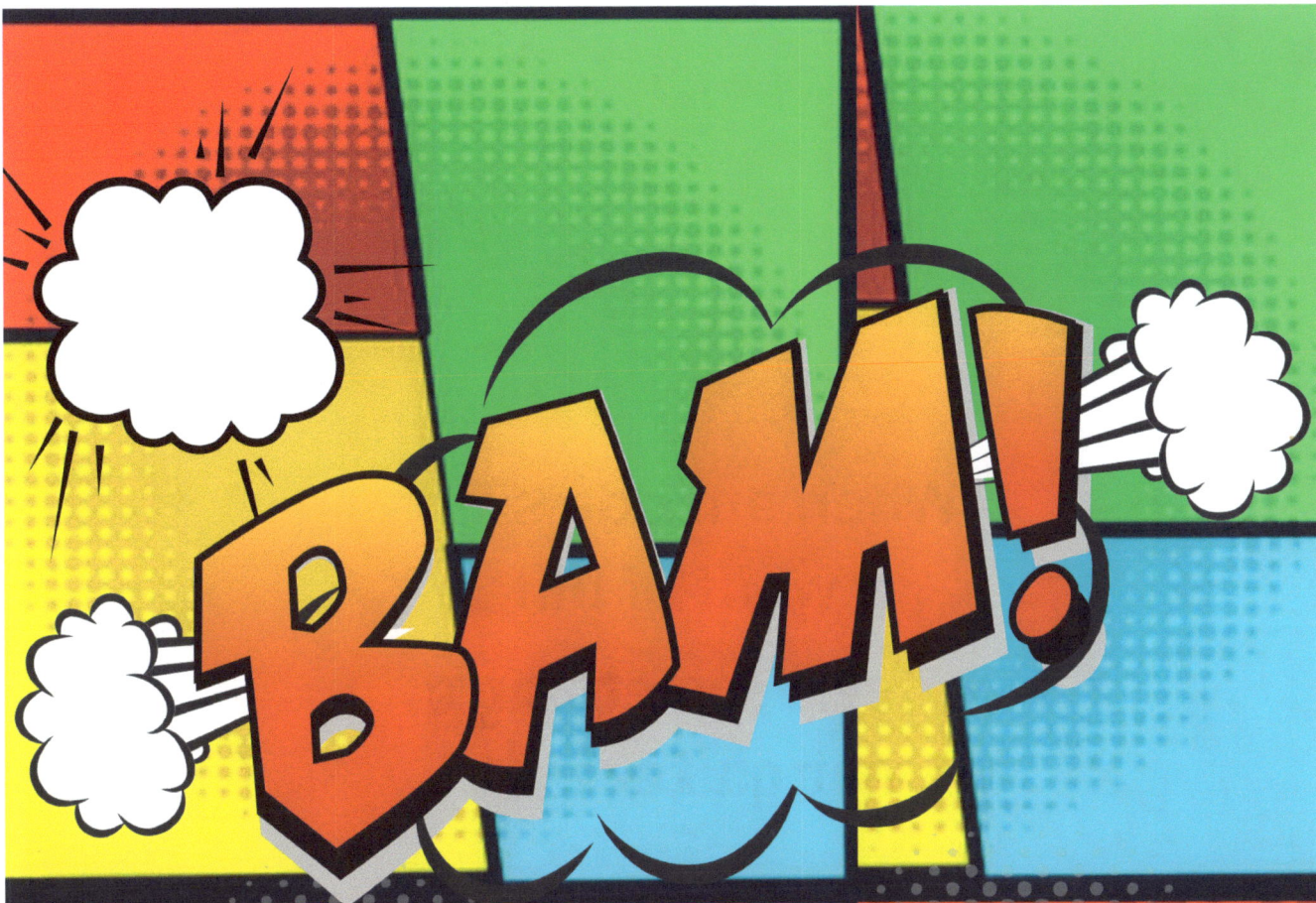

2
Fight Flight

When amigda sniffs
a whiff of biff ...

feels something's
not quite right ...

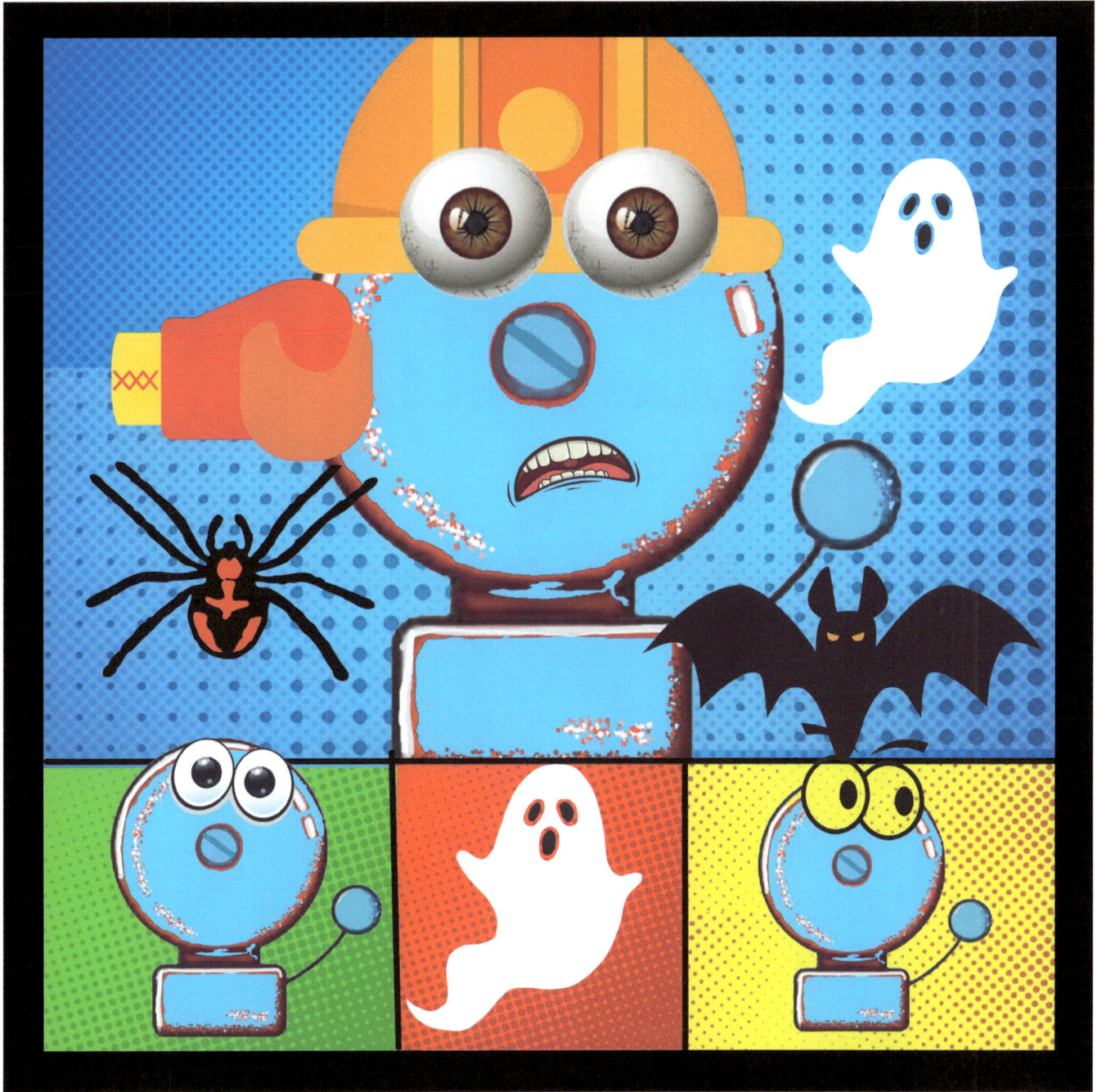

It activates survival
mode with

fight or freeze or
flight.

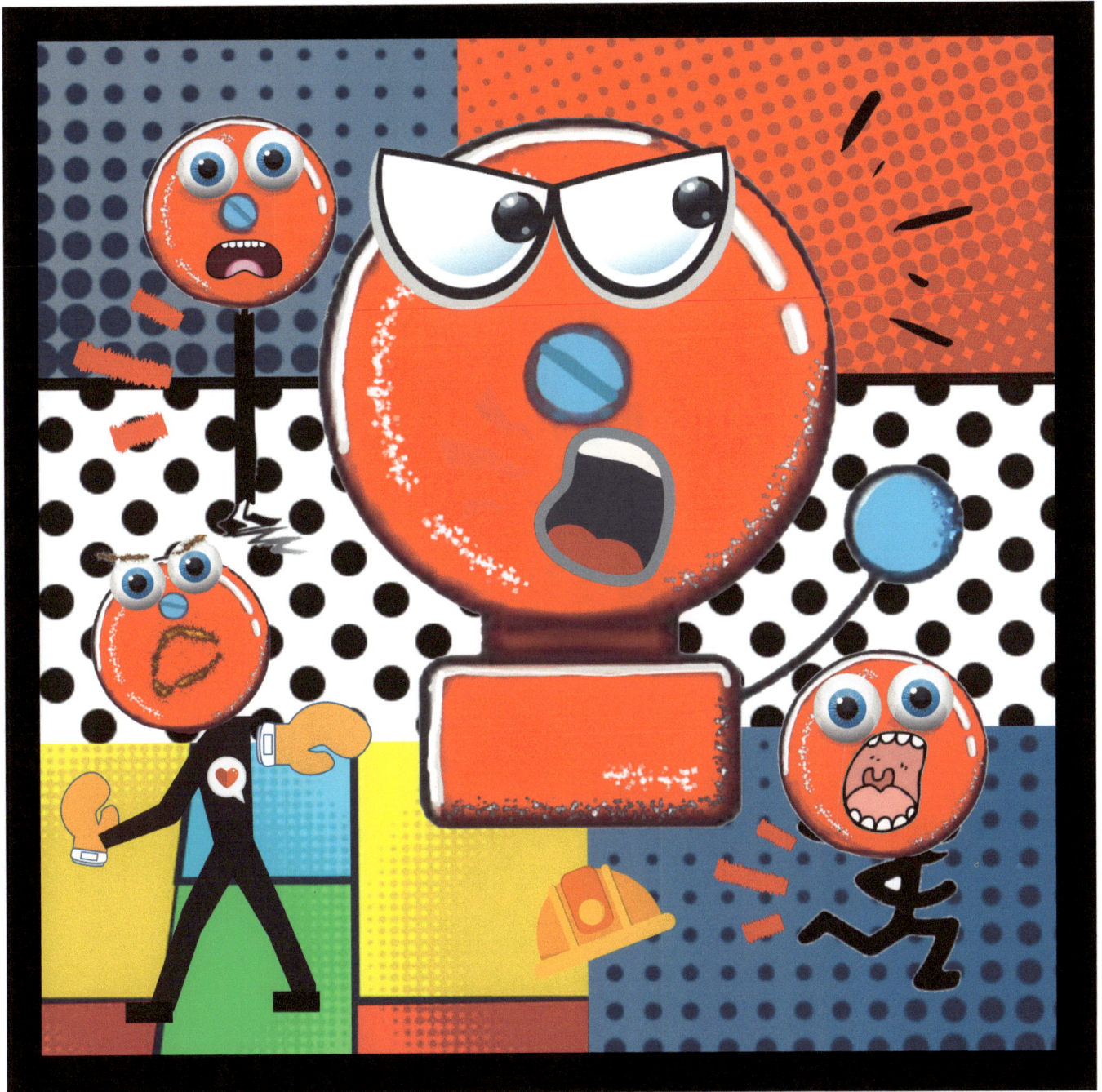

Zaps my blood with
strike-force chemicals
and shouts:

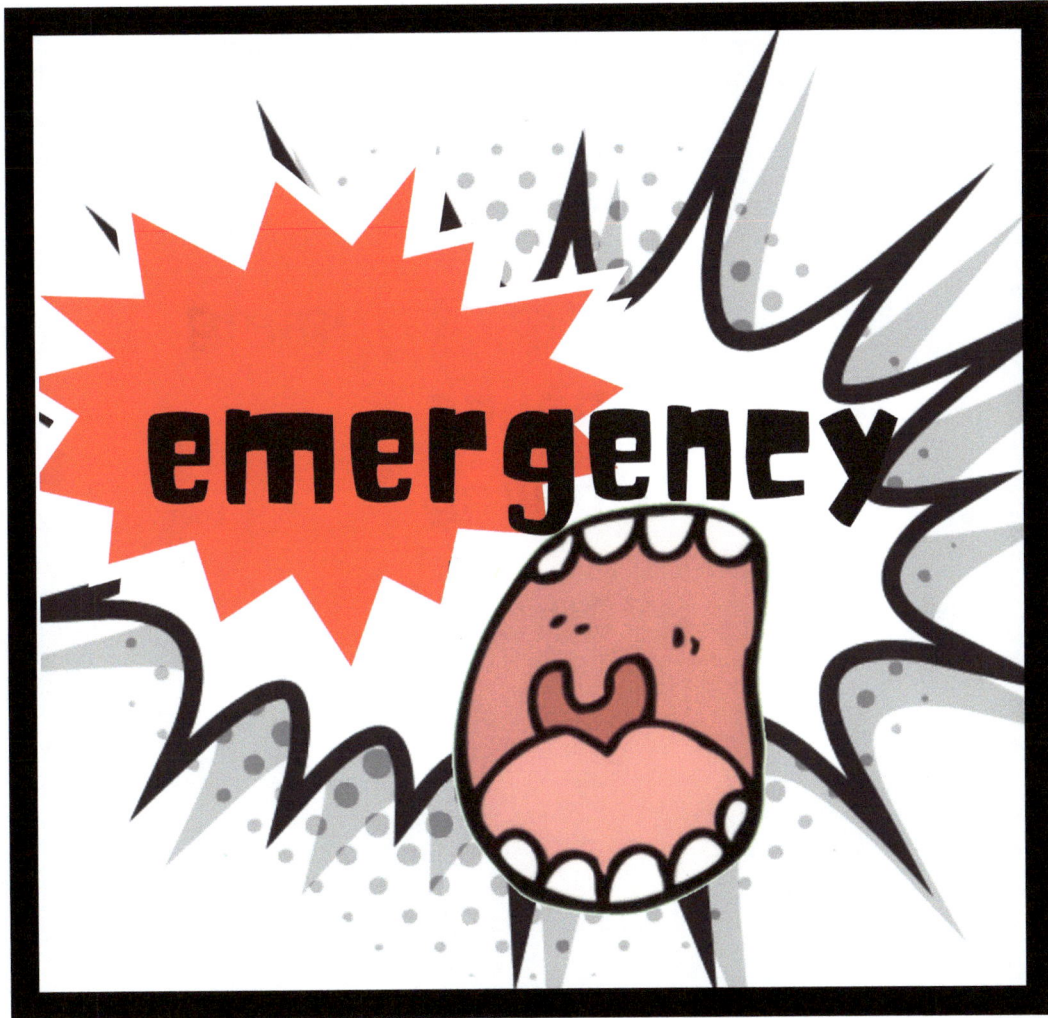

I'm in the grip of rippling,
crippling
trippling

urgency!

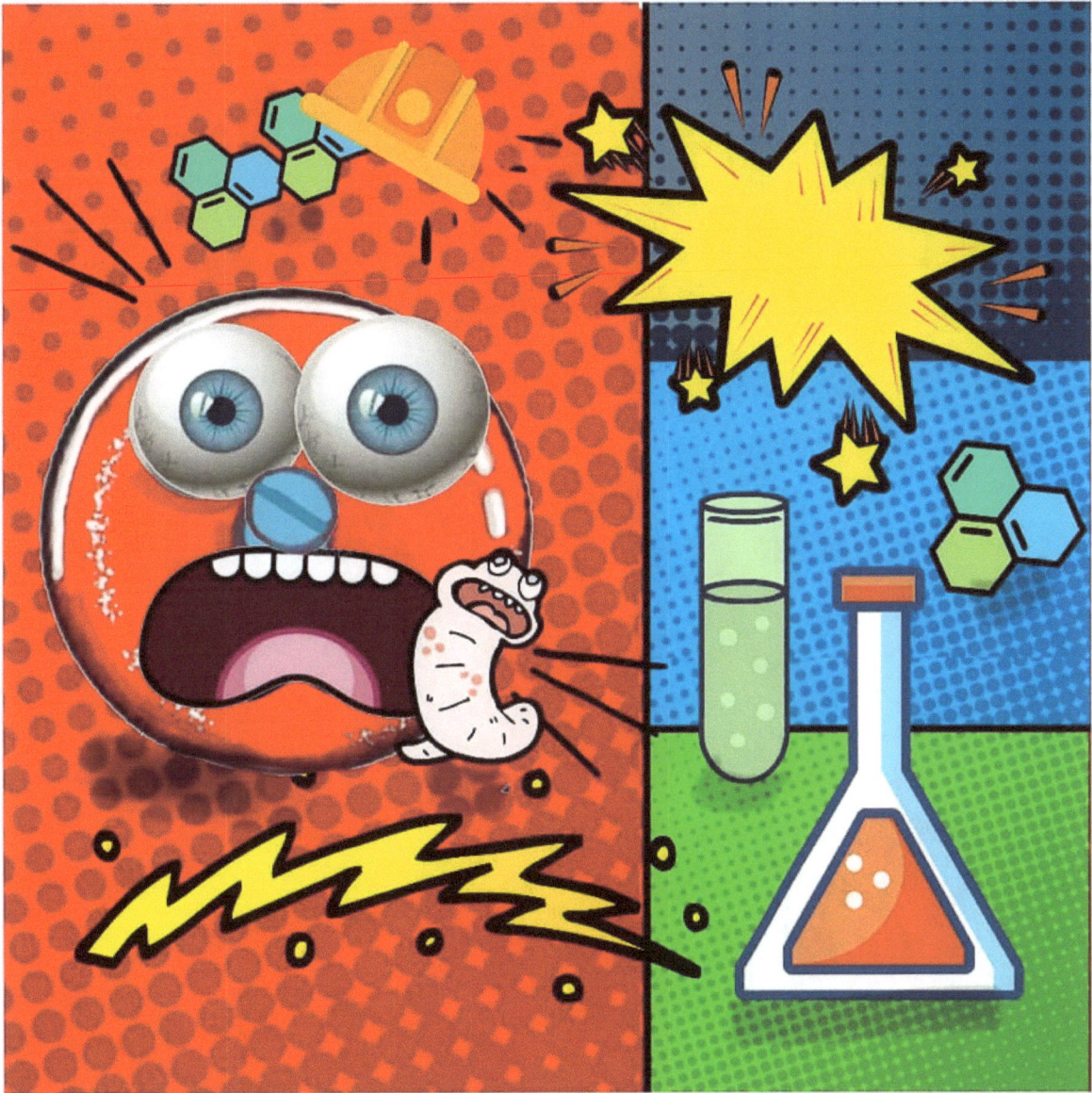

AMIG AMIG AMIG DA
la la la la, la-la

fight, flight, freeze, agghhh!

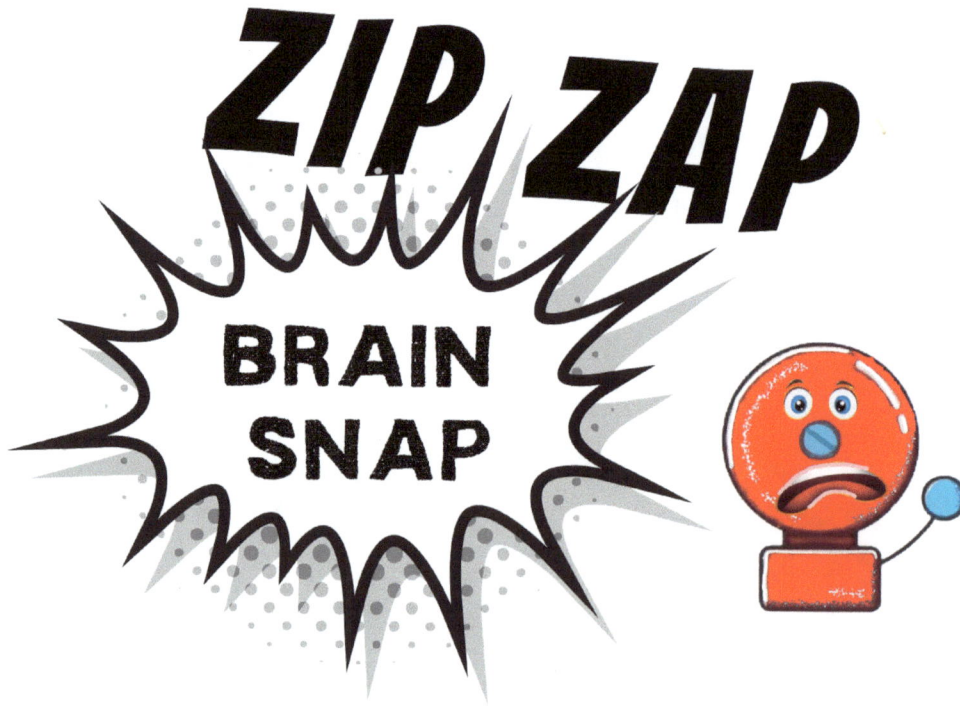

ZIP ZAP

BRAIN SNAP

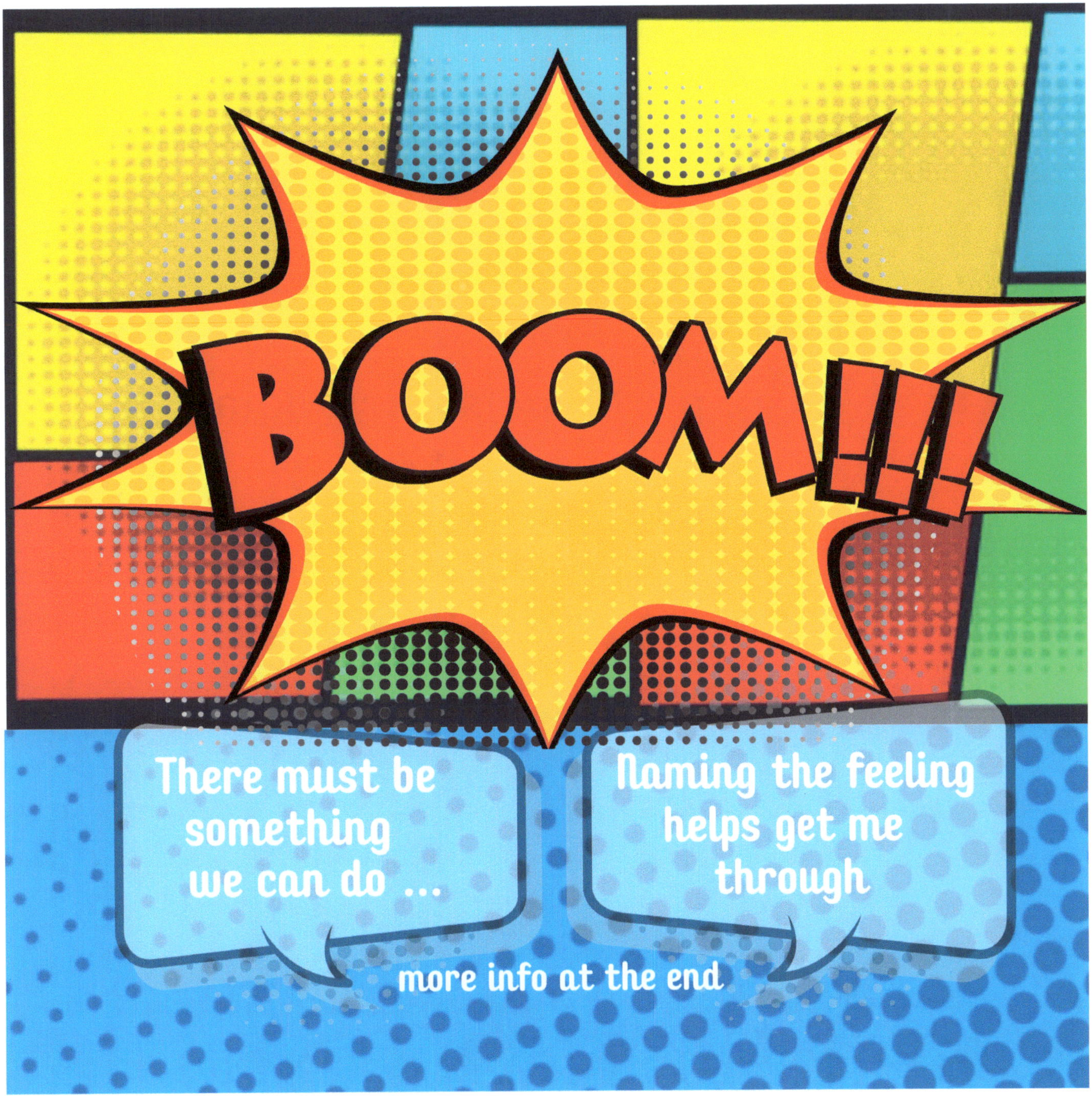
BOOM!!!!
There must be something we can do ...
Naming the feeling helps get me through
more info at the end

The problem is amygdala
does not really "get"
the difference
'tween a threat that's real
and routine small upset.

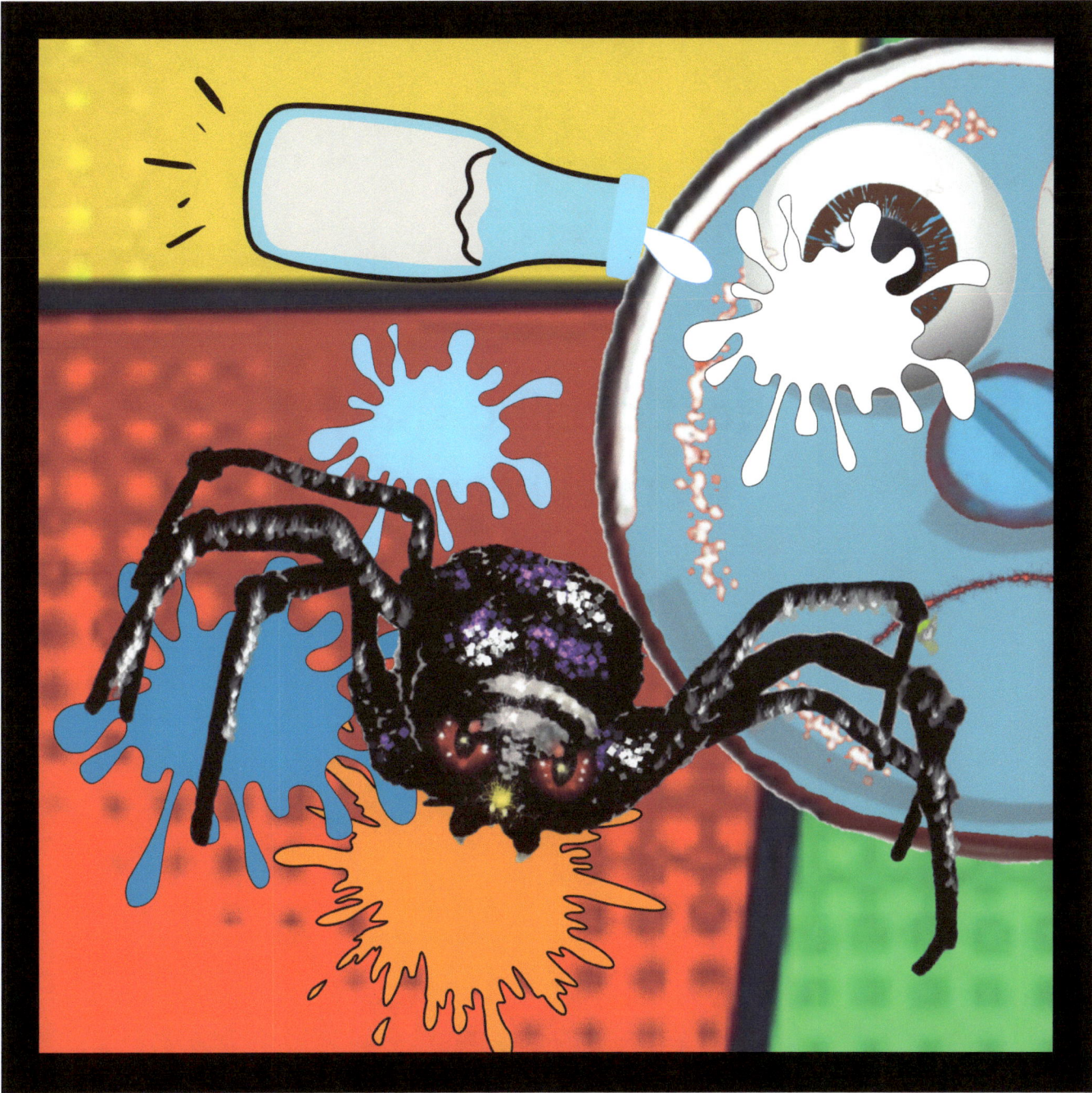

Be it circling shark,
a cruel remark,
lost keys or online hater:

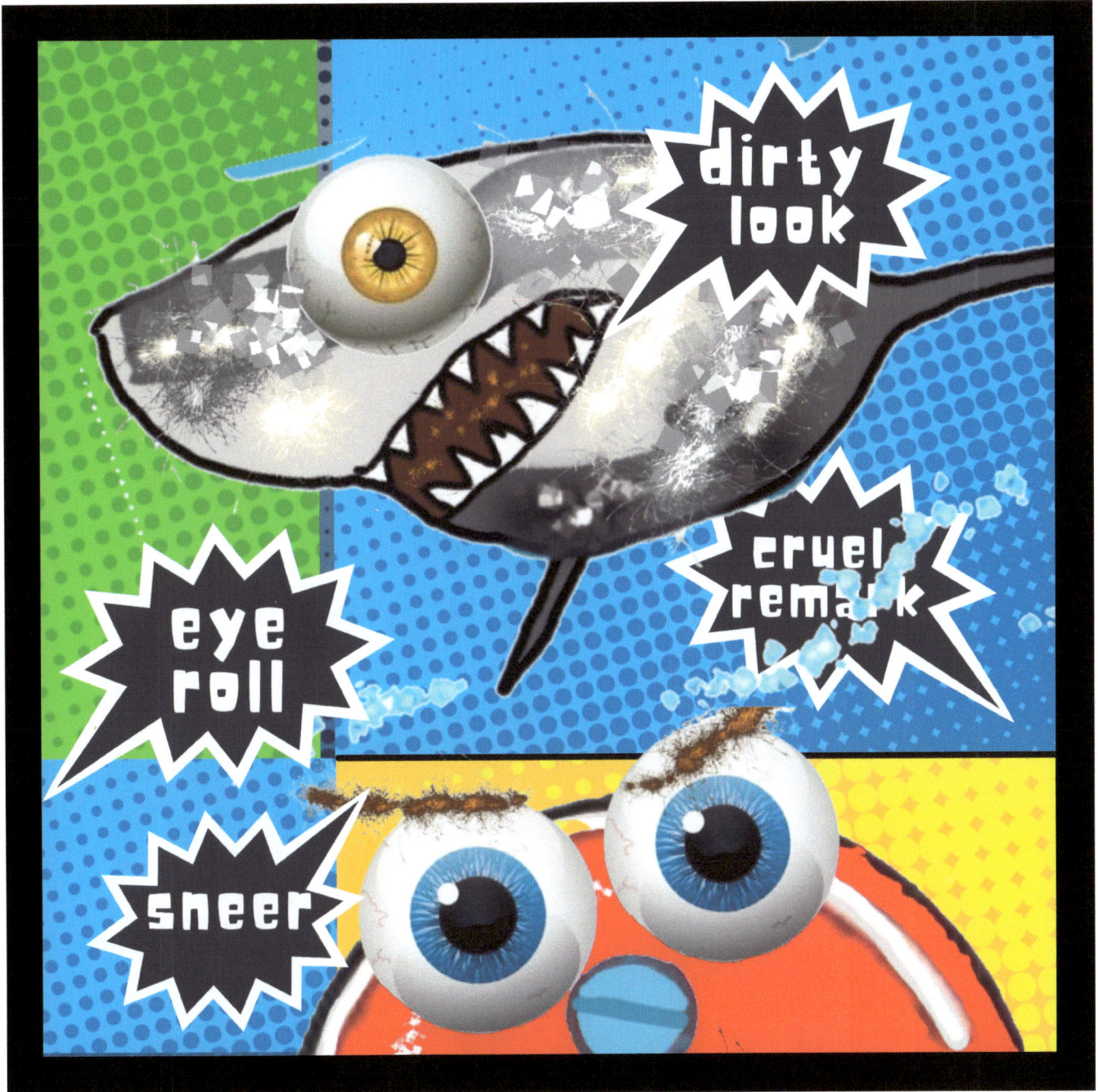

No time to think,
we're on the blink:

"Act now,
you can think later!"

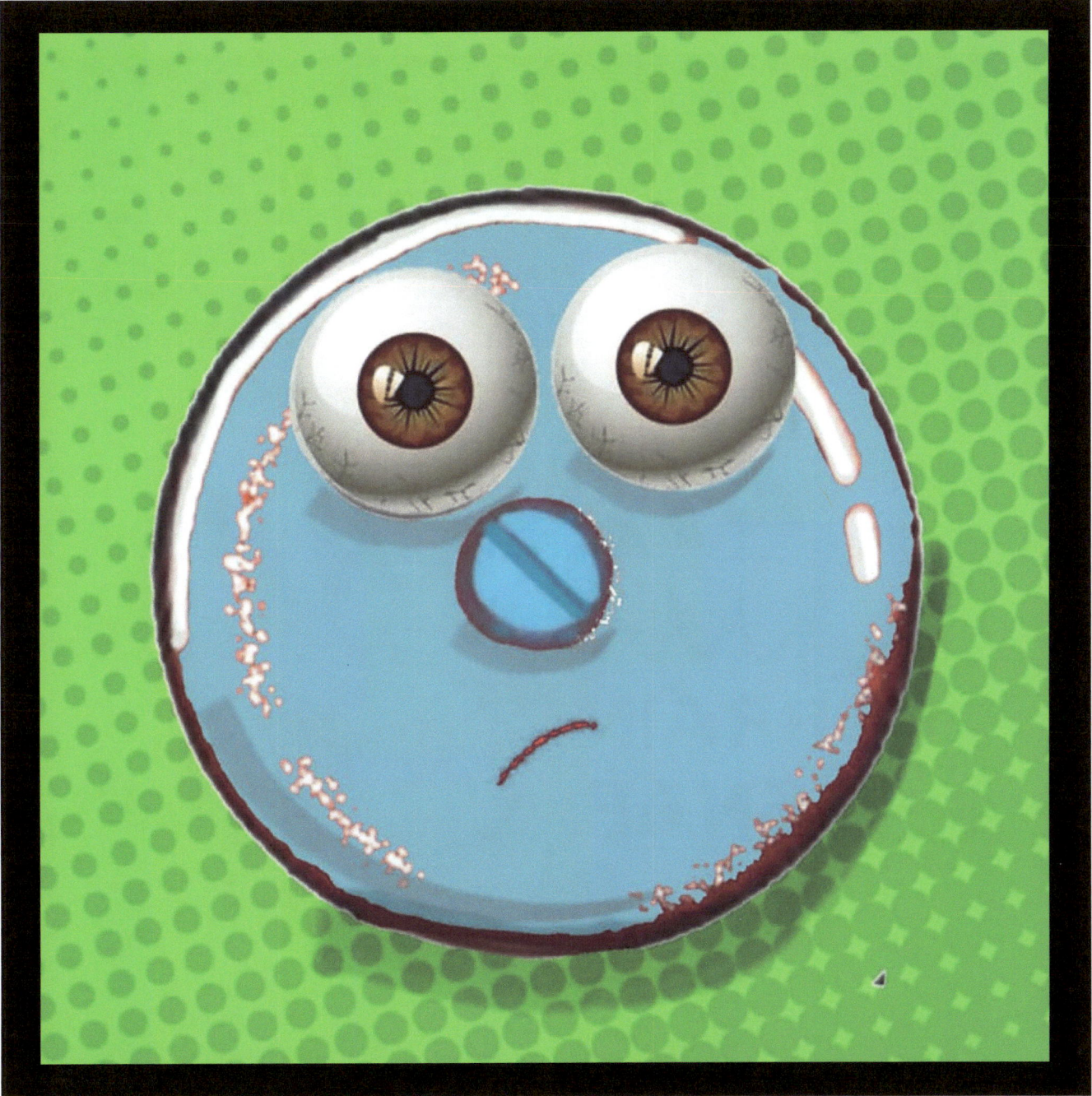

AMIG AMIG AMIG DA
la la la la laa-la

QUICK QUICK QUICK QUICK !

ZIP ZAP

BRAIN SNAP

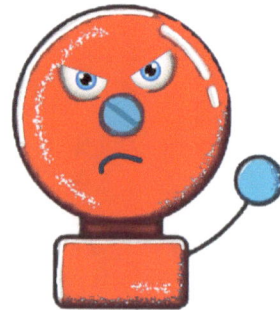

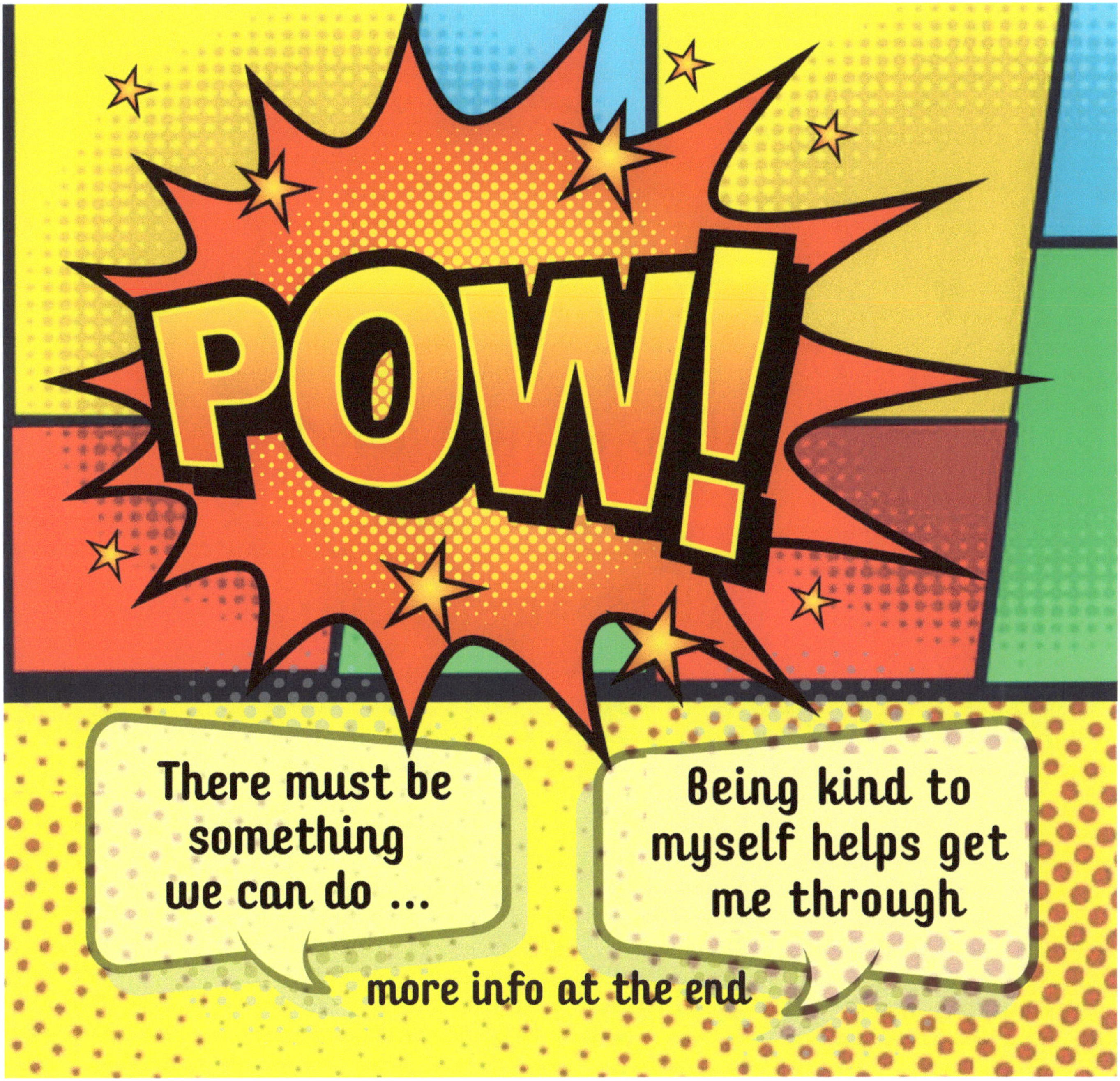
POW!
There must be something we can do ...
Being kind to myself helps get me through
more info at the end

Although we've left
the stone age

far far far behind

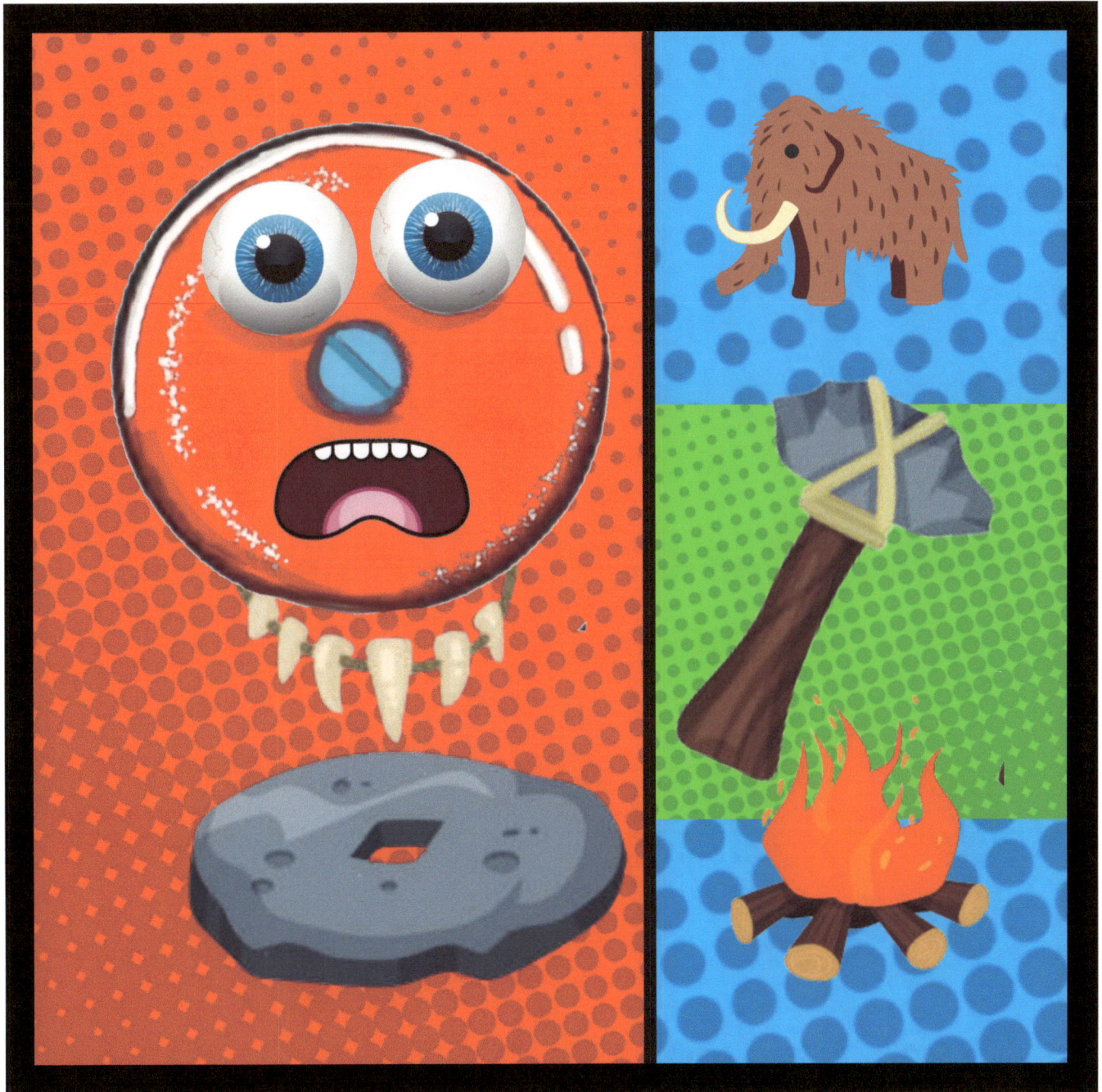

... the nervous system
still imprints
behaviours of a kind

meant for fleeing fearsome tigers,
meant for fighting
mighty foe.

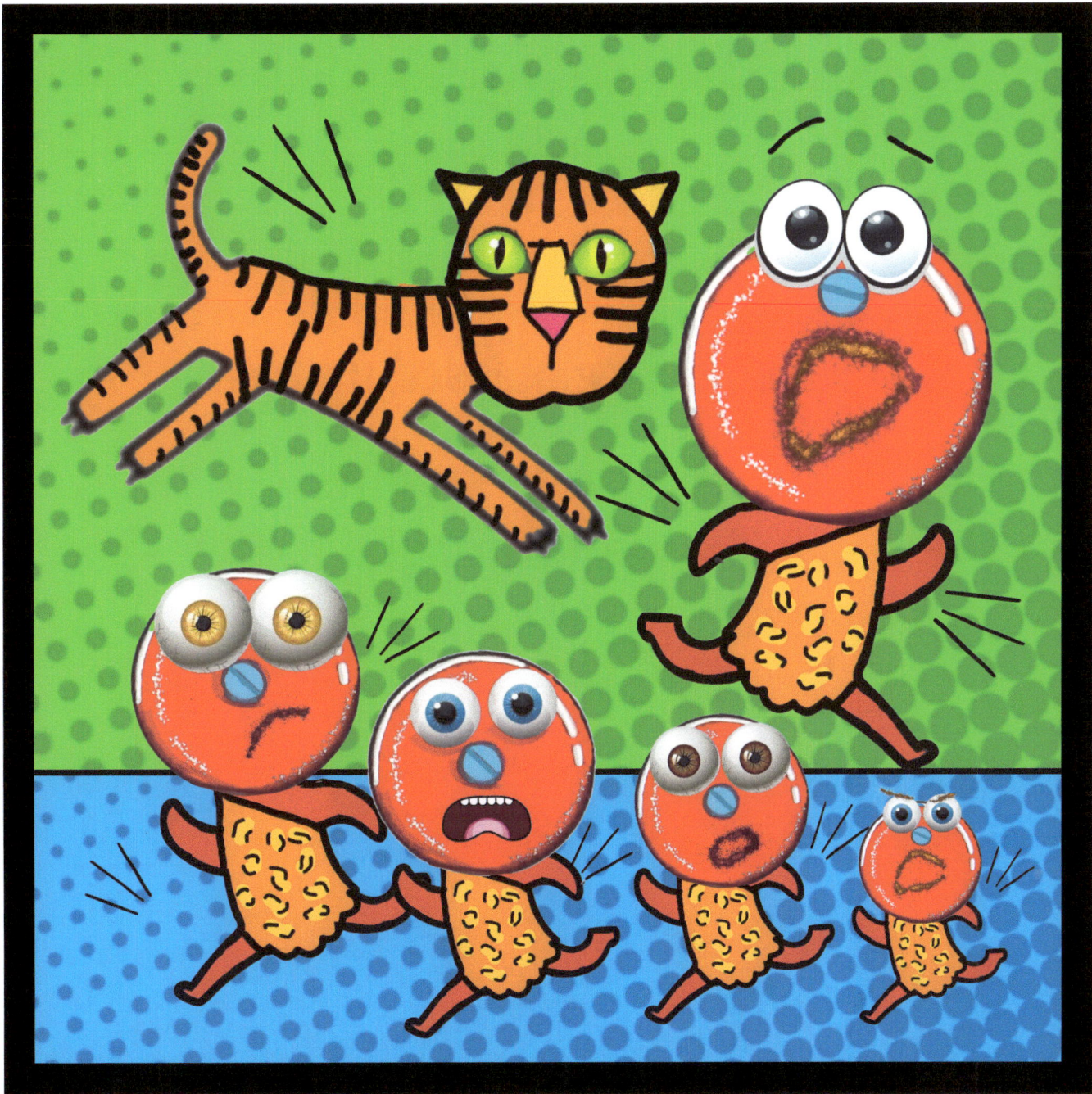

Today we're messed up by

the daily strains
we undergo.

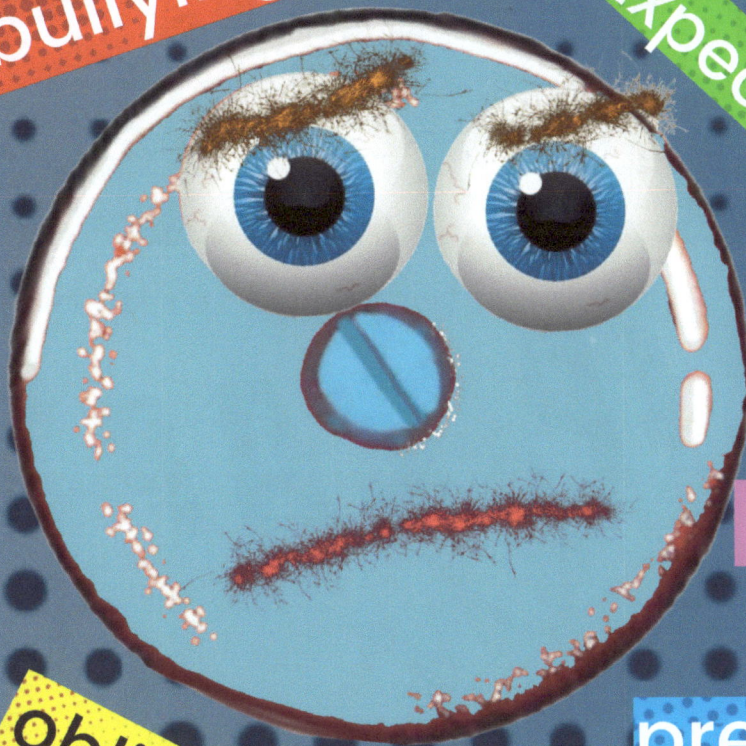

AMIG AMIG AMIG DA
la la la la laa-la

Hard-wired to over-react

ZIP ZAP

BRAIN
SNAP

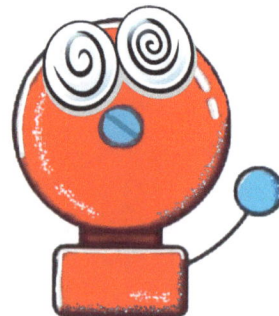

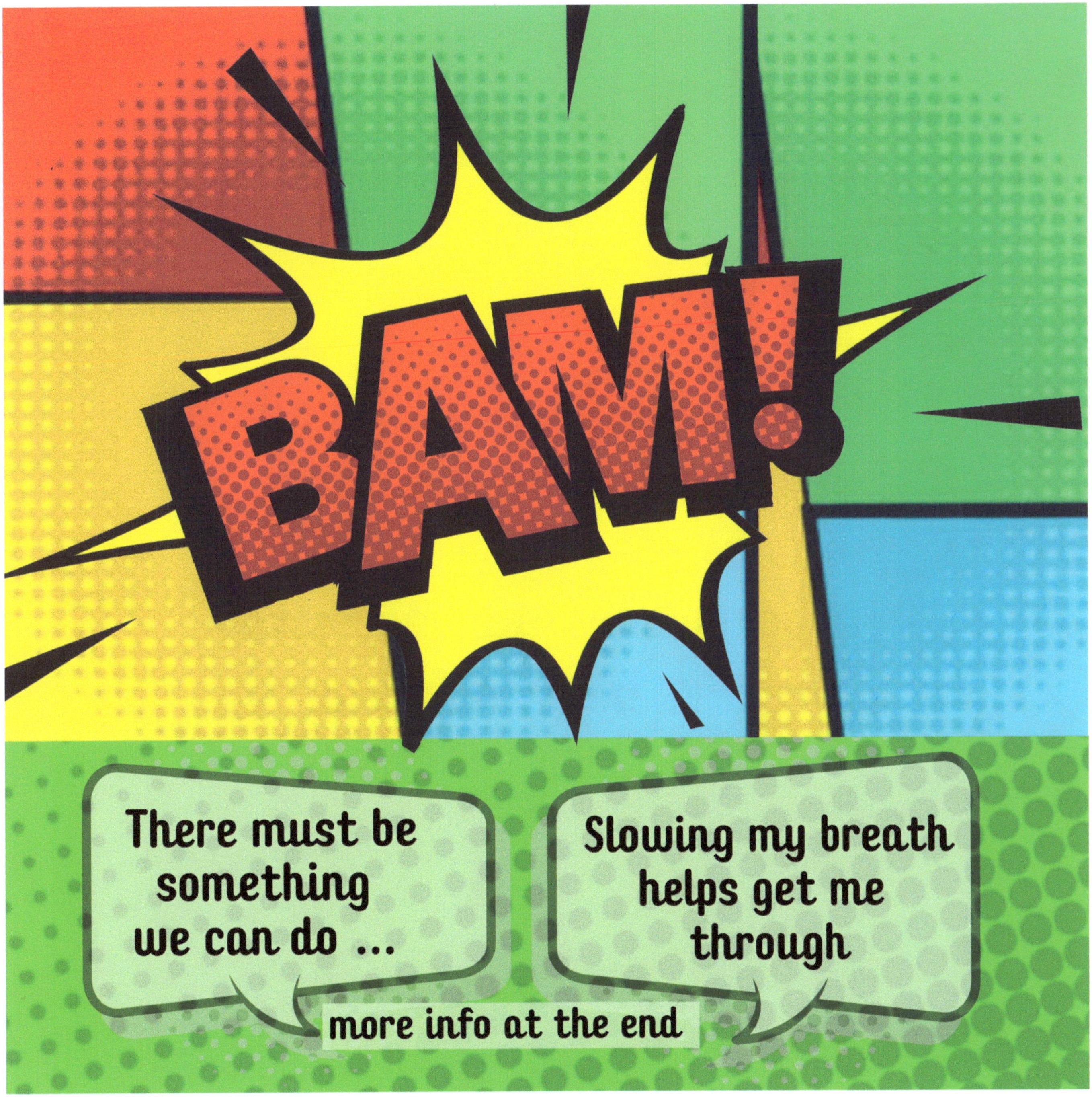
BAM!
There must be something we can do ...
Slowing my breath helps get me through
more info at the end

5
The Smart Part

The problem when amygdala
is bouncing off the chart,

it barricades the access to
my brain's best smartest part.

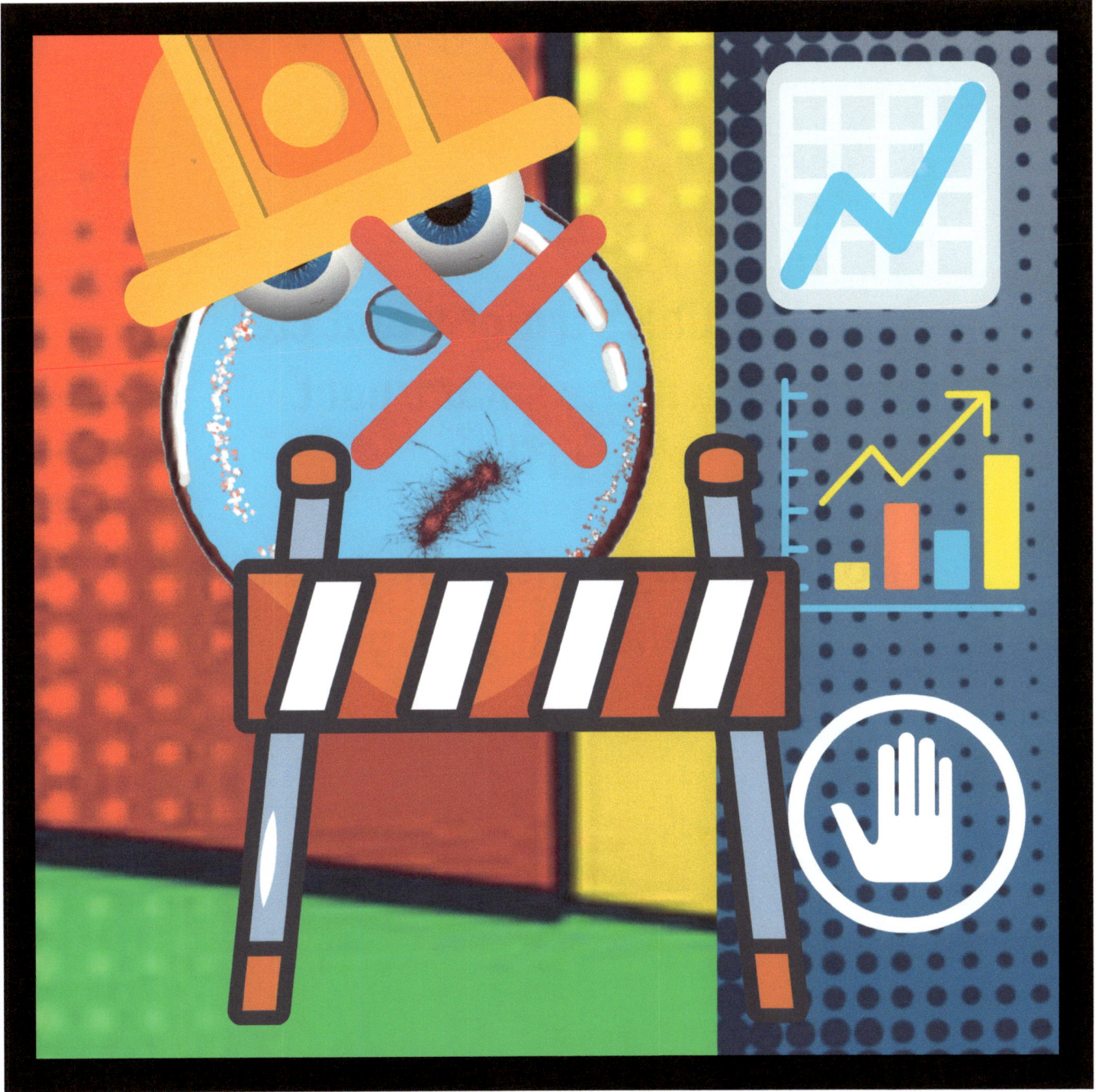

I can't think straight and clearly
when the smart part
is offline;

no pathway to its good advice,
intelligent design.

smart part

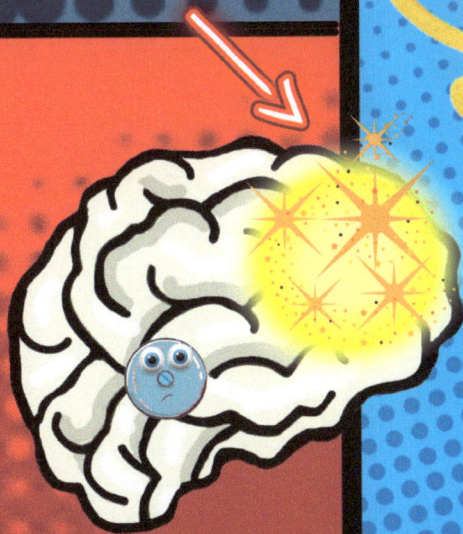

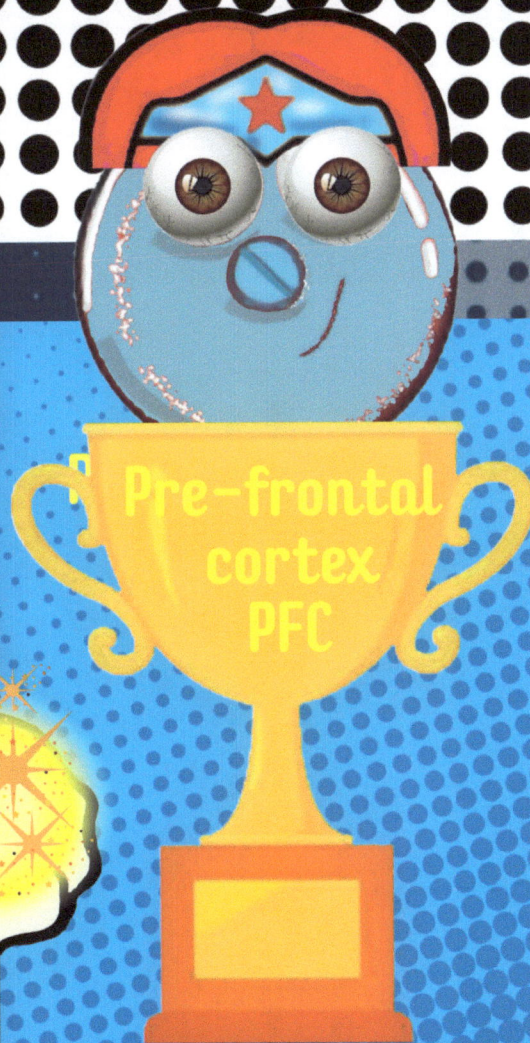

Pre-frontal cortex PFC

AMIG AMIG AMIG DA
la la la la laa-la

Pre-frontal cortex goes offline

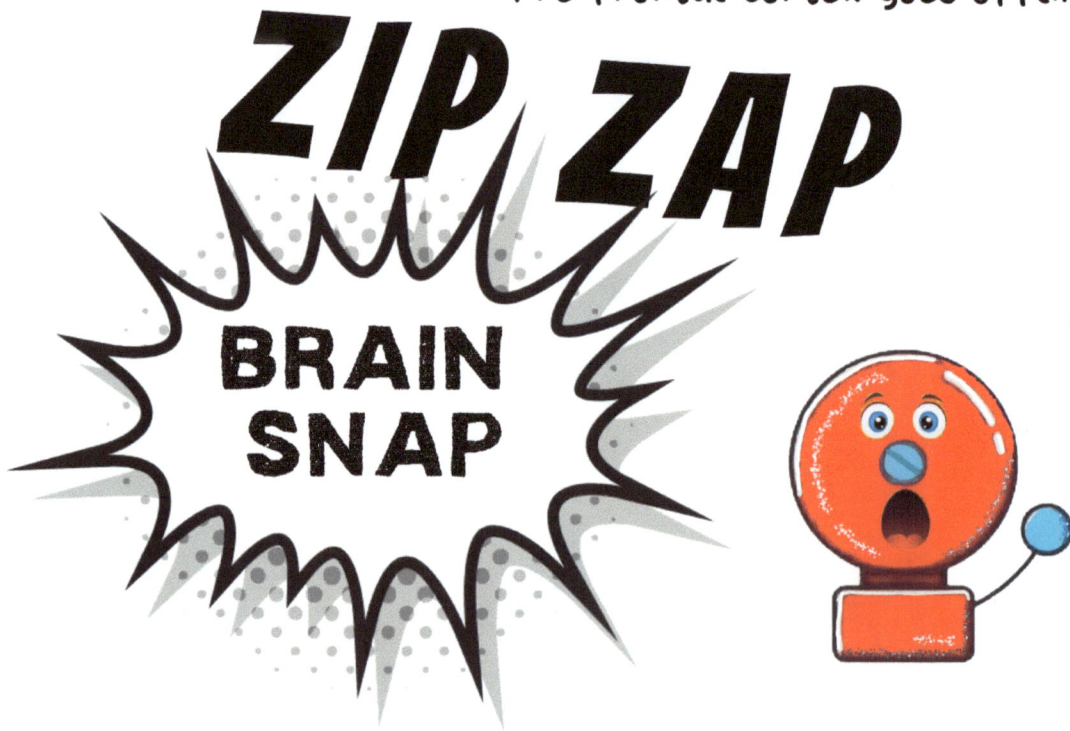

ZIP ZAP

BRAIN SNAP

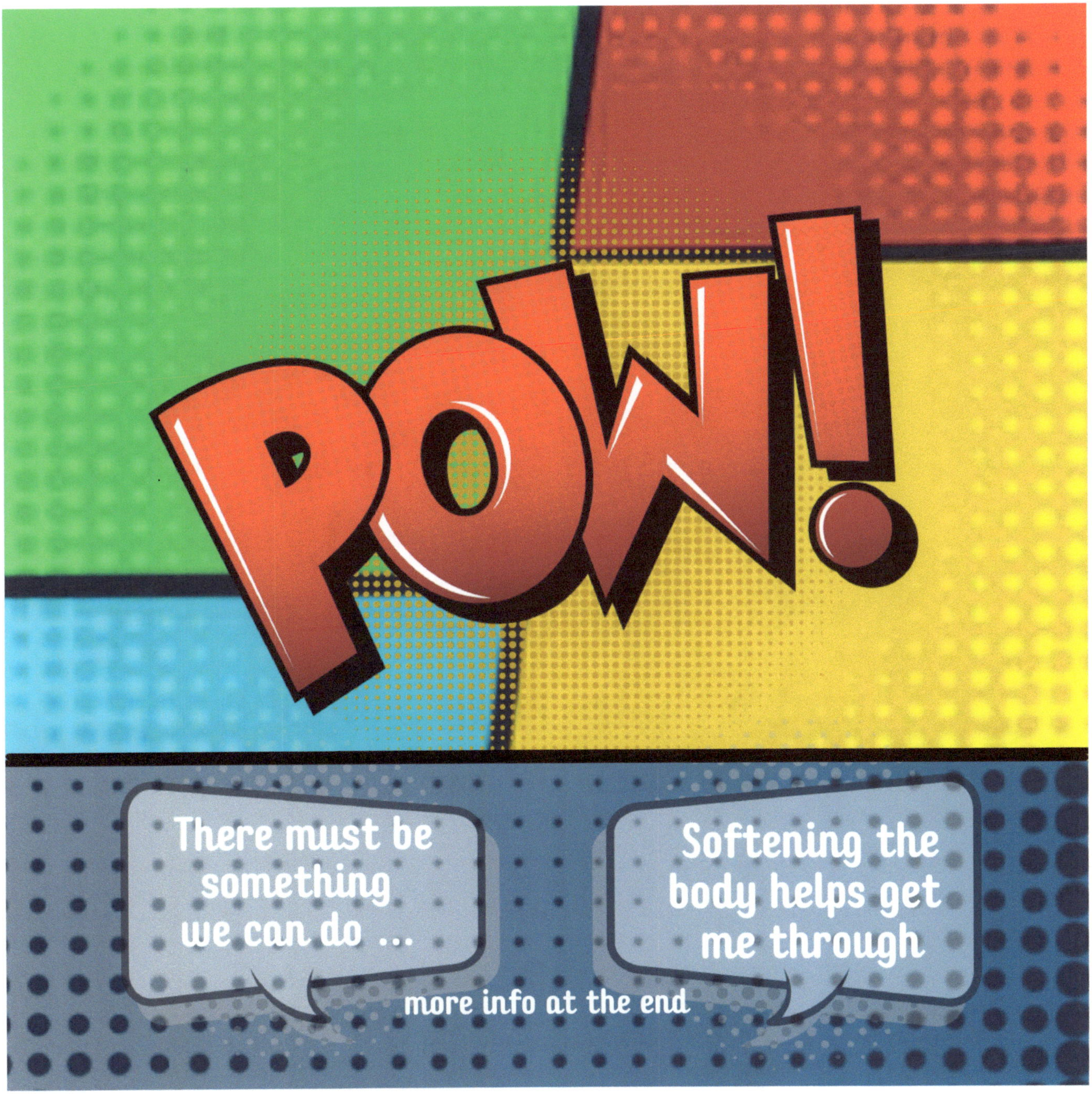
POW!
There must be something we can do ...
Softening the body helps get me through
more info at the end

6
Hard-wired

The trouble is amygdala
fires up all by itself;
it's hair-trigger activated

not a choice I make myself.

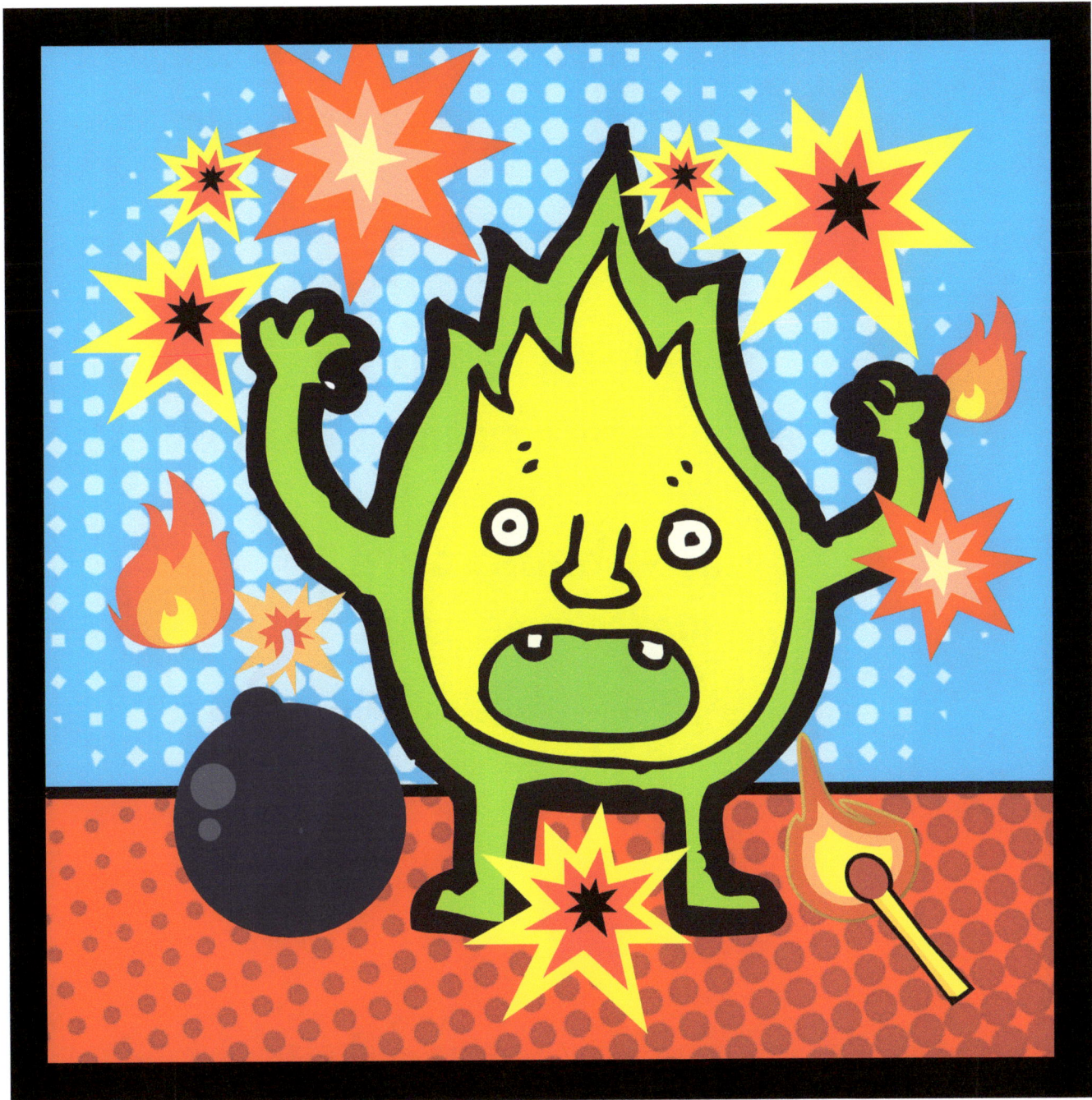

There's no course,
download resource,
sign-up, subscribe, submit or tender.

Just being born
makes me a pawn
in 'migdala's agenda.

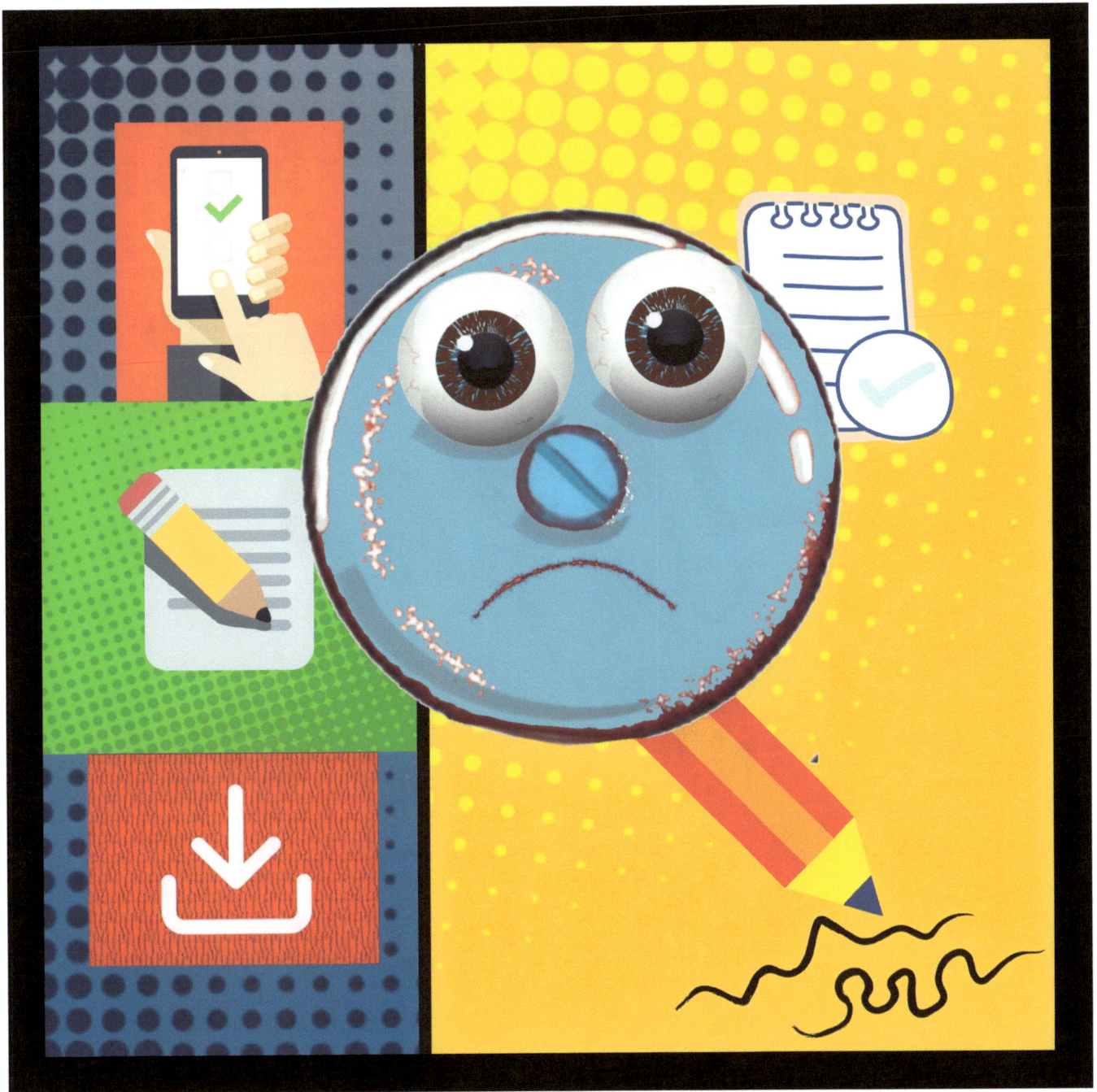

AMIG AMIG AMIG DA

la la la la laa-la

It's not your fault!

ZIP ZAP

BRAIN SNAP

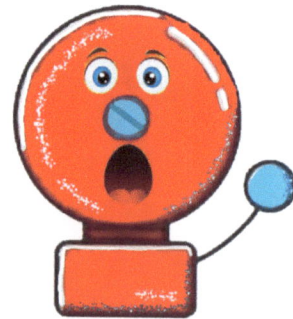

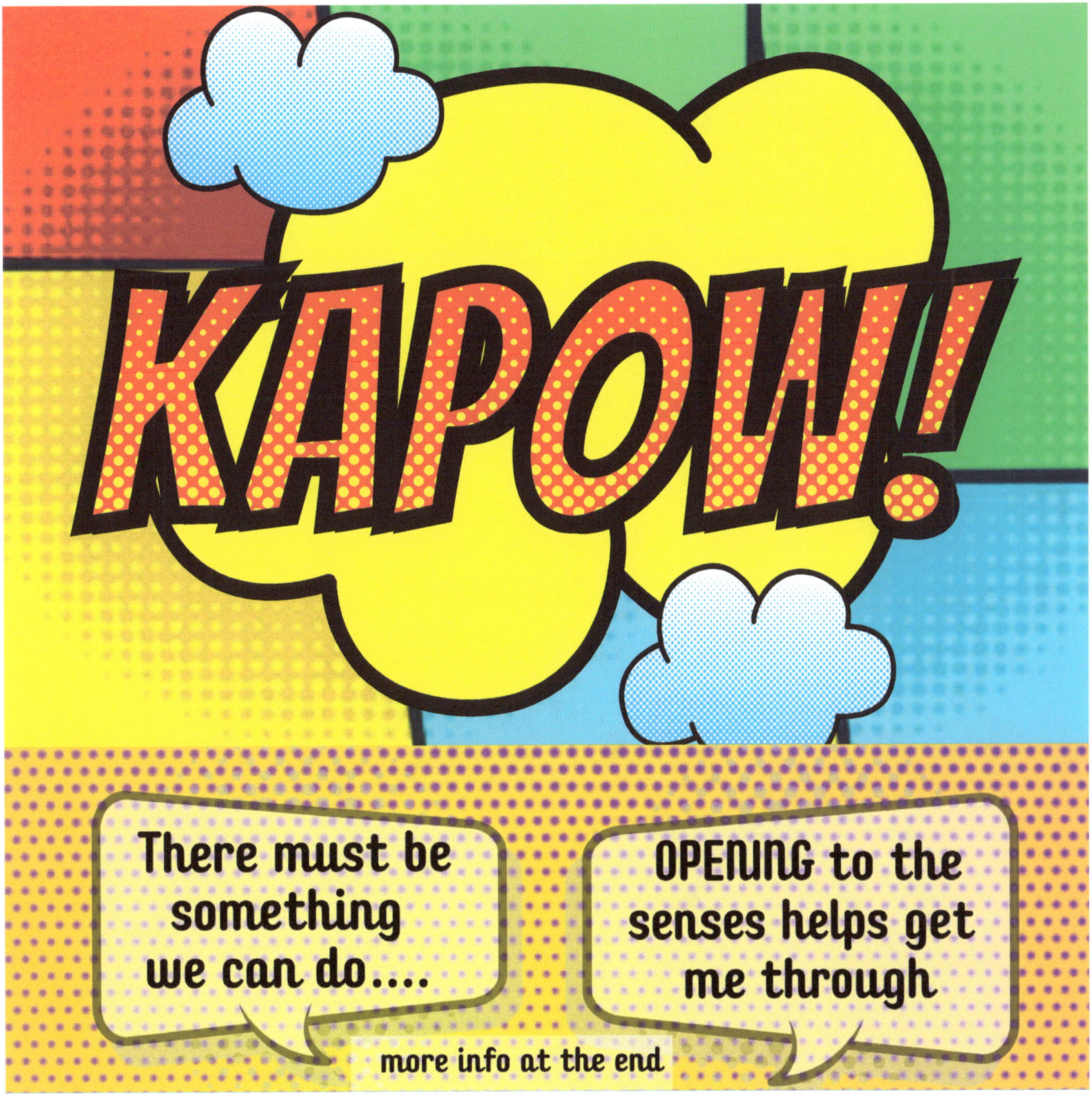
KAPOW!
There must be something we can do....
OPENING to the senses helps get me through
more info at the end

Have you noticed, sometimes noticed
how this happens in your life?

How you can't think
straight or clearly
when you're stressed
and under strife?

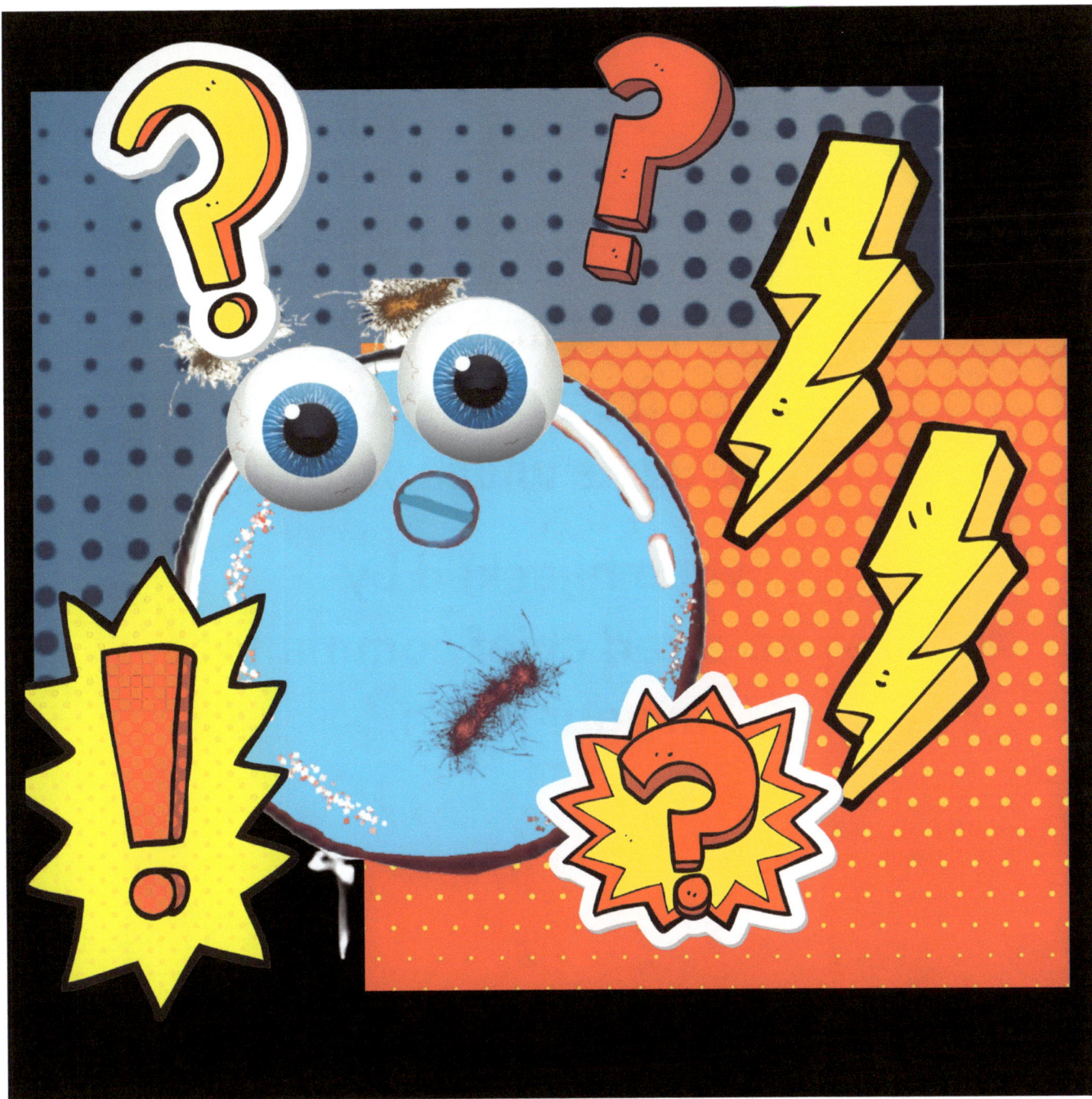

How you want to fight
or freeze or flee
or struggle under strain,

when hijacked by
the pea-sized chief commander
in your brain.

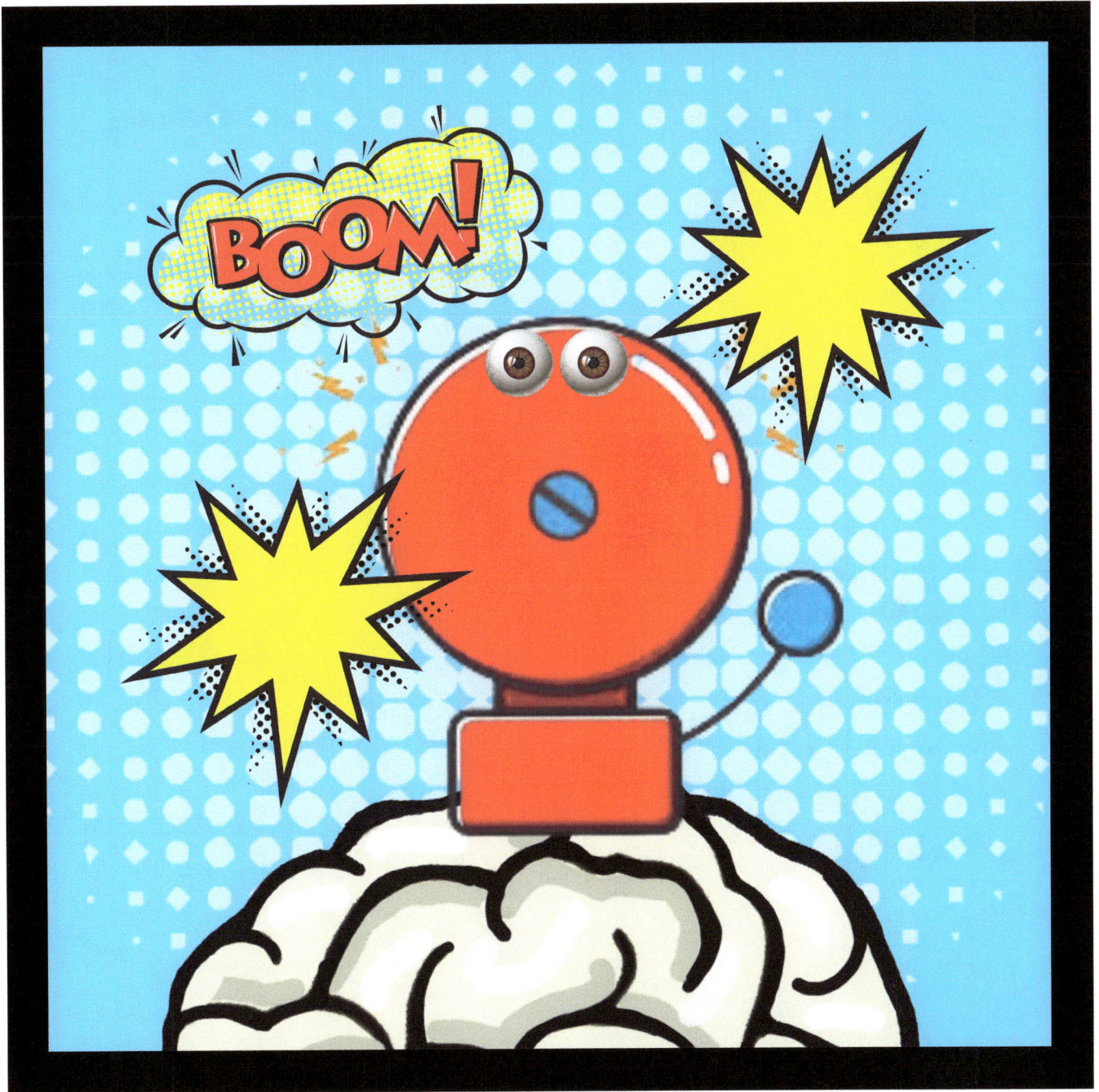

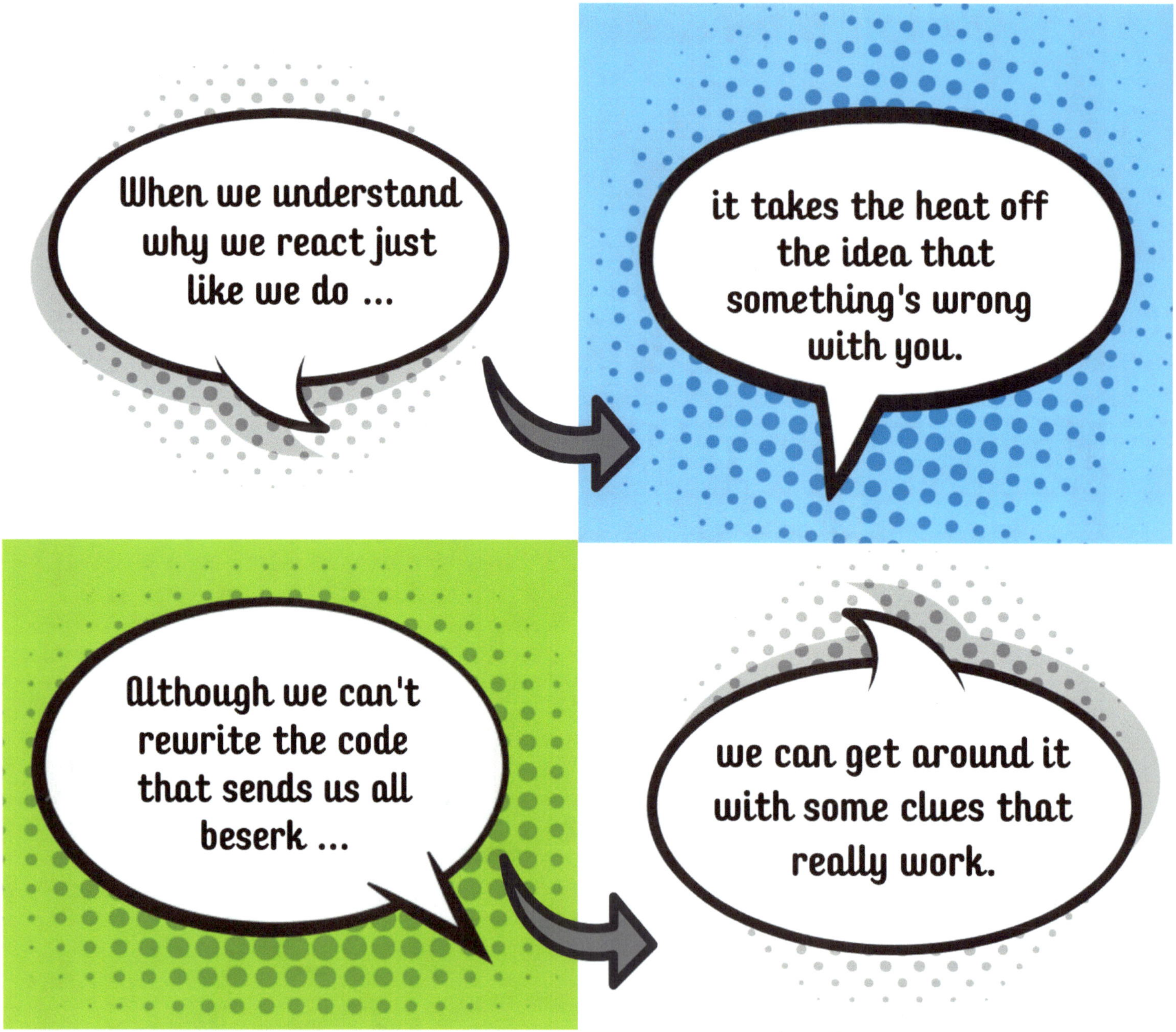
When we understand why we react just like we do ...
it takes the heat off the idea that something's wrong with you.
Although we can't rewrite the code that sends us all beserk ...
we can get around it with some clues that really work.

read on for

Six
clues to
defuse

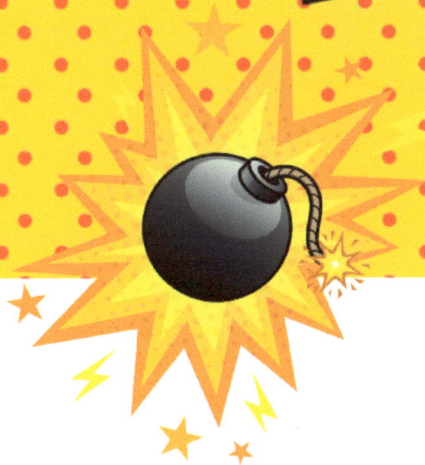

1.

There must be something we can do ...

NOTICING that I'm triggered helps get me through

Noticing versus switching off

It's important to notice the sense of being
triggered while it's happening.
Instead we often dive into fear, push it away,
pretend it's not happening
... none of which helps.
Instead, try allowing the experience to be there.
Releasing struggle helps calm the amygdala.
Then engage the next steps.

*In the case of trauma, please seek professional help.
(see page 61)

There must be
something
we can do ...

NAMING the feeling
helps get
me through

Naming is Taming

When you notice your amygdala is
triggered it's great to NAME your emotion.
"anger" ... "belittled"
"betrayed" ... "left out" ...
Clinical studies with people hooked up to
brain-imaging equipment show that
naming emotions calms the amygdala.

3.

There must be
something
we can do ...

Being KIND to myself
helps get
me through

Be kind to yourself

The powerful factor of self-kindness is often overlooked when we're stressed and upset.

Try treating yourself like you would treat a good friend or child in your situation. You're not being a sissy ... you're being human.

Self-comfort releases feel-good neurochemicals and switches off amygdala activation.

Go a step further ... imagine and empathise with other people in the same boat. Empathising with others helps us feel less isolated.

4.

There must be something we can do ...

SLOWING the breath helps get me through

Regulate your breath

The breath is not just for breathing. The breath taps directly into the nervous system. Deliberate regulation of breathing calms the amygdala.

Try counting to 5 on the inhale; 5 on the exhale. Then slowly extend the exhales to make them a bit longer than the inhales.

There must be something we can do ...

SOFTENING the body helps get me through

Soften your body

Stop for a moment and feel into
your body.
Notice if you are tensing anywhere;
soften through those places. Take your
attention around the body, soften any
tight places, soften any holding-on.

Softening the body calms the amygdala.
Soften as you breathe out.

6. There must be something we can do....

OPENING to the senses helps get me through

Connect to your senses

What can you see in front of you?
What do you see around you?
Or hear? Smell? Taste? Feel?
Activate whichever sense is easiest
to tap into right now.
Connecting with a sense dials down the
busy mind and calms the amygdala.

*A note about trauma

The trauma response is our evolutionary survival wiring. Nobody chooses it.

Post-traumatic stress disorder (PTSD) and chronic stress intensify amygdala activation. The amygdala tends to be more sensitive in an anxious brain.

When deep trauma and strong fear are present, proceed carefully if directly opening to the distress. Please seek support through a helpline or mental health professional.

61

Further reading

The MindUp Curriculum: Brain Focused Strategies for Learning. Grades PreK-2, Grades 3-5, Grades 6-8. The Hawn Foundation, Scholastic. 2018

Rick Hanson, *Buddha's Brain. The Practical Neuroscience of Happiness, Love, and Wisdom.* (with Richard Mendius) 2009

Dr Russ Harris, *The Happiness Trap: How to Stop Struggling and Start Living: A Guide to ACT.* 2008

Dr Jon Kabat-Zinn, *Full Catastrophe Living: How to cope with stress, pain and illness using mindfulness meditation.* 2013

Bessel van der Kolk, *The Body Keeps the Score: Brain, Mind, and Body in the Healing of Trauma.* 2015

Peter A. Levine, *Healing Trauma: Restoring the Wisdom of Your Body.* 2019

Richard C. Miller, *The iRest Program for Healing PTSD.* 2015 (book and mp3 audios)

Kristin Neff, *Self-Compassion: The Proven Power of Being Kind to Yourself.* 2011

Kristin Neff, *The Mindful Self-Compassion Workbook* (with K. Germer). 2018

Dan J. Siegel, *The Whole-Brain Child.* 2018

Also by Shakti A. Burke

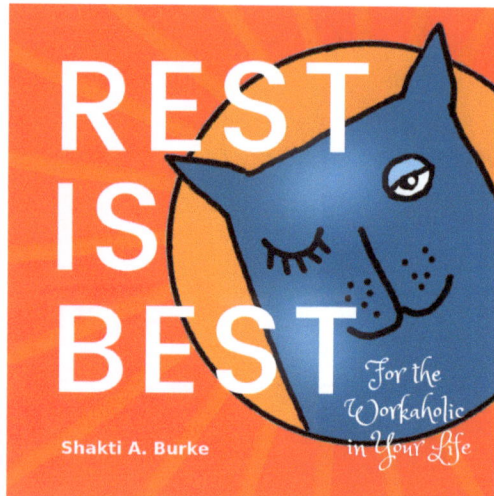

Be inspired to live the good life through the power of rest! Let's face it, overwork leaves little room for living the life you want. Regular rest strikes the balance between ease and the effort/exhaustion treadmill. Light-hearted verse and images lead you through this warm, inspiring picture book aimed at the workaholic in your life!

Available at Amazon, booksellers or joyfulmind.net.au.

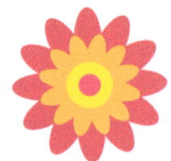

Please visit www.joyfulmind.net.au for Shakti A, Burke's mindfulness blog, and information about her online courses and local classes.

Sarvam mangalam "May all beings be happy"

joyfulmind.net.au